Your Face After 30

Your Face After 30

The Total Guide
to Skin Care and Makeup
for the Realistic Woman

Jan Hayes-Steinert

Illustrations by Glory Brill Schmerzler

A & W Publishers, Inc.
New York

Published by
A & W Publishers, Inc.
95 Madison Avenue
New York, New York 10016

Library of Congress Catalog Card Number: 78-53066
ISBN: 0-89479-015-3

Designed by Fran Miskin
Printed in the United States of America

To my toughest critic, my husband, and for Laurie and Larry, and to my first inspiration, Bette, and my ongoing inspiration, Bea.

Acknowledgments

To the physicians and dermatologists who checked my work for accuracy, my utmost thanks. For professional and ethical reasons their names may not appear here.

To Elaine Markson, my literary agent, who paid me the supreme compliment of saying "yes" within twenty-four hours.

To Jane Toonkel, my acquiring editor, who possesses a directness and decisiveness that is truly a joy to work with.

To Paul Fedorko, Angela Miller and Lesleigh Lad, who were supportive and instrumental in the completion of the book.

To Glory Brill Schmerzler, my illustrator, who interpreted every idea and rough drawing into just terrific artwork with her amazing ability to crawl inside my head.

Contents

Introduction 1

PART I You and Your Skin 11

Your Skin 13
Makeup? Anything is Easy When You know How! *14* • What Is
A Good Makeup? *15* • A Dressing Table? *16* • Truly Essential
Beauty Tools *16*

Your Skin Structure 21
Your Natural Protection *23* • The Effects of the Sun on Your Skin
Structure *25* • Preventive Care Means Protection—Protection
Means Preventive Care *29*

Skin Types: Are You Really Sure of Yours? 31
Skin Types *33* • Black Skin *39*

Cleansing Your Skin 43
#1, You *43* • Cleansing Cream or Lotion *44* • Soap and Water *47* •
Your Precious Eyes *57* • Skin Fresheners *58* • Moisture...
Moisturizers...and Moisturizing *61* • Night Creams and Lotions
65 • Disciplining Yourself! *69*

Daily Cleansing Procedures 71
A Few Words About Products *71* • Oily Skin *72* • Normal
Combination Skin *73* • Dry Skin *78* • Very Dry, Sensitive or
Delicate Skin *80* • Ultra-Dry (Dehydrated) Skin *82* • Three-Minute
Nightly Action Capsule *84* • Supplementing Your Skin's Cleansing
Program *85* • A Special Note to the Mature Woman *89*

Special Facial Beauty Procedures 91
Let's Have A Clear Understanding of Blackheads, Whiteheads
and Pimples *91* • Action Capsule *99* • Eyebrows *101* • Action
Capsule *104* • Action Capsule *109* • Facial Hair *109* • Facial
Exercise *113* • Neck Exercise *114* • Old Standbys: "Frownies,"
Chin Straps and Headbands *115* • Cosmetic Surgery *116* •
Allergies *123* • Commercial Vs. Homemade Products *126*

PART II Makeup 127

Makeup! The Excitement Begins 129
Who Makes the Best Makeup? *131* • How to Put Different Type
Products Together *133* • Balance and Harmony *134* •
Contouring *138* • Face Shapes and Hairstyles *150* •Tinted
Foundation for a Natural Look *158* • Blusher or Rouge *167* •
Eyebrows Reflect Our Character! *173* • Face Powder *178*

Eye Makeup: Every Woman Is An Artist! 184
Individualized Eye Makeup for 25 Eye Shapes *186* •
Eyeshadow *200* • Eyeliner *203* • Eyelashes *206* • A Word Of
Caution *215* • Good Makeup and Precious Time *215* •
Eyeglasses *215*

Lipstick Was Born in America in the 20th Century 221
The Better Way to Better Lips *225* • Correcting a Not-Too
Perfect Mouth *227*

Teeth 233

Last Words 235
Your Accessories *235* • Manners and Makeup *236* • How to
Approach A Cosmetic Counter *237* • Makeup Action Capsules:
Daytime Complete Makeup *238*; Quick Getaway Makeup
240; Evening or Gala Complete Makeup *240*

Index 243

Your Face After 30

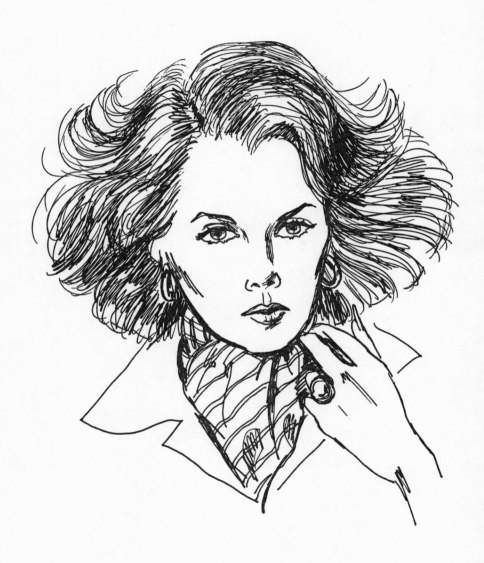

Introduction

YOUR FACE AFTER 30
AND THE REALISTIC WOMAN

Women, by nature, are realistic. It is an inherent trait in most all women. The word *realistic,* itself, means different things to many people. Whatever meaning it may have for you, I think you would agree that it has a positive connotation. You would say to yourself, "yes, this word describes me." Realism is an area where we women score points well above the opposite sex.

To me, one of the foremost meanings of the word *realistic* is common sense. It is my feeling that if you explain something simply and clearly to a woman, although she may not agree with you entirely, she will apply her own good common sense to that subject. She will delete what does not appeal to her, and apply the rest to her way of thinking and style of living.

We are living in an age, especially now, when we don't want to be told just what to do—we also want to know why we should do it. And there must be a good reason if we are expected to comply. Dictates of any kind are out! We no longer accept the dictates of fashion designers. Fads are not a must—they are only for those who want to wear them. The "in" thing is to be yourself and to appear natural. And isn't it about time?

There are many books on the subject of beauty, all very much alike in their appearance and approach. All very lovely to look at and fun to thumb through but, frankly, on behalf of women everywhere I am tired of their complicated texts, confusing illustrations, flowery language, and color pictures of gorgeous women.

1

Most realistic women cannot personally identify with actresses, models or members of the jet set even though it is amusing to read the gossip about these people, and heaven knows we need heroines. But most women know instantly that they could never look like the picture of the beautiful model or glamorous star. They feel defeated before they have started, therefore many don't even try.

This book concentrates solely on the subject of your face and will not delve into other beauty areas such as the bath, nails, exercise, diet, and so on. It is not cosmetically complex. I feel that most women would rather have an intensive course on one subject on which they can concentrate, than a little bit of knowledge on each beauty subject covering the body from head to toe. While that type of encyclopedic beauty book serves a purpose, women generally don't learn very much that they can actually use to enhance the beauty of their own faces.

There are certain areas concerning faces that have been "closet" subjects up to now. These topics are often either deliberately neglected or have been lightly skipped over, leaving you discouraged and confused as to what personal course of action you should take. We are going to discuss such subjects as blackheads and excess facial hair in full detail, and decide what methods are the best for each individual woman.

Even with the new found knowledge and methods for self-application that you will find in this book, there may be certain areas of advice that are not for you. Only you can decide! Some women simply cannot make use of any corrective beauty treatment and should instead see a dermatologist (a doctor who specializes in skin disorders and diseases). Throughout the pages that follow, you will be advised where and when this is the best course to take.

Mainly, we shall deal with what are considered minor and superficial skin problems in relatively healthy women. These problems are not disorders or diseases. It is not my purpose to provide do-it-yourself data in the area of medicine. When and where cosmetology encroaches on medicine and the medical profession, you will find that I distinctly draw the difference.

Cosmetic plastic surgery is a subject many women have on their minds these days and this, too, we shall discuss from a woman's psychological point of view. And, as almost any doctor will tell you, the psychological relationship between appearance and mental health has long been established.

Another comment is in order: While it was not my original intention to mention products by brand name—I am not a spokeswoman for the cosmetic or toiletries industry—I find I must put some of these products (though by no means all) into categories. Otherwise this book would be incomplete and most certainly less useful to you. The motivation for this book was my hope to banish confusion and remove the mystique associated with certain products.

Many of the products I mention by name are selected by you, the consumer, in the supermarket or in a self-service store without benefit of behind-the-counter advice. Others are not, but I do not intend to circumvent the lady behind the cosmetic counter—the consultant, demo, beauty advisor or cosmetician. She can be an indispensable friend to you and your beauty needs. Usually she is well intentioned and deserves your confidence.

In writing this book, I find I am in the fortunate and unique position of being beholden to no one other than myself. I was formerly employed in an executive marketing capacity as well as being involved in many other areas of the cosmetic industry. When one is currently employed in any capacity within this industry, and is writing about it, "certain considerations" regarding products and practices—whether they be omissions or glorifications—are inevitable. These considerations cannot be avoided and undoubtedly would affect me as well, if I were still connected in any way with the business. Nor do I take the position of scandalizing or being an inside informant, as many other beauty book authors have done in the past for the sake of sensationalism. If you are looking for villains, you will not find them here. Individual villains do not truly exist. In fact, the real villain is the confusion that abounds about products and their usage. My research has led me to an in-depth study of this subject and I have found confusion to be prevalent in the minds of women everywhere.

While it is not my motive to enhance the image of the cosmetic industry, I must say in all fairness that it is very good about being a self-regulatory industry—certainly head and shoulders above the food or automotive industries, which more readily distribute their products with known hazards. There are such isolated cases by minor cosmetic manufacturers. However, I know conditions to be hospital clean where products are compounded and packaged. Quality control all at all stages is effectively and consistently employed by most manufacturers. Only recently, I was invited to inspect a large, modern facility where all conditions could have met the standards required for the site of a delicate heart transplant operation, and this is indicative of all the manufacturers mentioned in this book.

Instead of scandalous gossip or inflated egos of the beauty business and its' individuals in this book, there will be truth and honesty about products, their reason for existing, the purposes for which they were intended, and their uses on your face.

SOME PERSONAL NOTES AND THOUGHTS

I literally grew up in the cosmetic business. At age fifteen, I started in the retail end of the beauty business with an after-school job. Within five years I owned my own shops with makeup artistry (my first love since the age of seven) as my specialty.

Disbanding my business a few years later, I went into the manufacturing end of cosmetics where I felt I could be more creative—besides, I really wanted to learn the business from the ground up, particularly product development and marketing. In the early 1950s Revlon afforded me this opportunity for they were eager to hire bright young women of executive caliber willing to work at the factories. A new campaign of "glamour" in the Revlon image was to be spread, and I was the initial secret experiment. The joke circulating around Revlon's Fifth Avenue office was that they had Suzy Parker working at the plant as well as in their advertisements. Indeed, my boss, Raymond Nash, the director of manufacturing, came storming in one day and in utter earnest said, "Since when are you modeling on the side? I thought I kept you busy enough." It was very flattering since Suzy Parker was the "face of Revlon" then, as Lauren Hutton is the face of Revlon's "Ultima" line today.

Nonetheless, I learned about production lines, components, raw materials, filling, packaging, batch production, lab testing, forecasting, purchasing, quality control, and a million other things. I returned to school and took specialized courses and seminars of all kinds. Some of the most famous people in various phases of the beauty business became my mentors. They said I had a "natural creativeness." I was eventually to prove it when many of my ideas were realized as products on the retail shelf and when models in magazines were using the "looks" I created with those products. Working my way up didn't happen overnight, however. I left Revlon to go on to Westmore, Kurlash, Fabergé, Coty, Lilly Daché, to list a few, and then back twice again to Revlon's Fifth Avenue office (known in the industry as the "revolving door").

While I loved it, I do have certain misgivings. Uppermost in my thoughts is that having been a part of this industry when women were wooed away from soap and water in exchange for cleansing cream, I now feel a tremendous sense of personal guilt, particularly when I look at the skin of today's over-30 woman. Her skin, and this may very likely apply to yours, has a much greater potential than is currently realized. Putting your best face forward is a series of details that builds to a final picture. Seemingly small details are all-important and "technique" in both cleansing and making-up has been the missing link up to now.

The techniques that appear in this book have been developed and tested by myself as well as some of the best experts in the field. While you may find some techniques contrary to what you have previously read or even used, I assure you they are the very best that modern research has brought to light, and, in most cases, it is the only way certain products will work together for the utmost effect while at the same time guarding and preserving your skin and, just as important, your eyes. I wear the entire spectrum of makeup every day of my life, not only because it makes me look my best, but when I look my best I feel my best. I am not alone . . . most realistic women will admit this is true. More and more, beauty is considered to be how we see ourselves, for we are constantly told that one does not radiate beauty to others unless one possesses self-confidence and emotional health to begin with. This is not a superficial veneer. Foremost psychologists tell us that "it is more important than our physical and material needs. The psyche requires a healthy vanity for an individual's general well-being."

In the immediate years after age 30, our faces reflect one of the best stages of life because the youth of the 20s still radiates while at the same time a certain knowledgeable look, gleaned from acquired wisdom and experience, accompanies it. If only more of

us could realize this wonderful mixture of youth and sophistica-
tion while still in our 30s instead of bemoaning our actual age,
we would appreciate and be happier with ourselves instead of
allowing society to place such enormous importance on chron-
ological years. Isn't it time we came to just that?

After 40, our faces can be even more beautiful; they display
the love and interest that has been developed and devoted to
others and ourselves, while attaining the deeper self-knowledge
that enriches one's personality. While we are not oblivious to the
fine lines that may be more noticeable at this stage of life, they
are inconsequential. Our positive actions and outgoing activities
make us feel younger and therefore look younger, and represent
genuine personal growth. While a woman's 40th birthday may
have made her feel it was the psychological dividing line between
youth and middle age, isn't it really to be considered a woman's
most active prime?

A woman's face after 50 is one of the most beautiful of all in
my estimation. It has arrived at a stage of contentment and satis-
faction and represents the willing spirit of what one has done
with one's life, the mistakes made and learned from, the reckon-
ings one has come to terms with. The experiences of life produce
a face that is magnificent in terms of one's acquired breeding
and one's infinite potential. After 60 is the culmination of all
these ages and phases and the face has a unique beauty.

The question raised here is: Where does outer beauty converge
with inner beauty? Should outer beauty be dismissed as irrele-
vant? Does it involve conceit or deceit? And how much importance should be placed on it? In my heart, I feel there is no
contradiction between these two kinds of beauty. They walk hand
in hand, and when we are at our most successful stage in life,
they emerge as one—fresh and unobtrusive. If any levelheaded
woman at any stage in life possesses the attributes of vitality,
unselfishness and compassion, she is motivated to greater heights
by first caring for herself. History has proven that this will always
be the first prerequisite. To be physically beautiful is rarely an
end in itself.

TO BEGIN WITH

This book was deliberately meant to be uncomplicated—to be used as well as read. It was designed to sit on your dressing table or wherever you make up to facilitate your using its instructions. To begin with, refer to the book often while you are in the process of making up. When you become adept and have mastered its information so that it comes to you automatically, referring to it will no longer be necessary.

I am sure, by this time, you have read many beauty articles with alluring and promising titles such as "Beauty is, as beauty does"; "Self-confidence is 90% of the beauty game"; "Sex is a must for the beautiful woman"; "Happy thoughts are beauty itself", etc., etc., etc. All this is true and contributes to you as a total person. But we are going to focus on the outer woman, for inner beauty is first reflected on our faces.

We will concentrate on you as an individual to make the most of each and every feature so that you evolve as the very best possible YOU. In the pages that follow you will learn about the structure of your skin, so that you have the working knowledge that you need. Technical names that you may have heard or read about will be enclosed in parentheses ( ), so that the association of terms may be planted firmly in your mind, if you wish to utilize them. This is by no means necessary! The illustrations that go with the text are accurate, in that they are medically based. They have been clarified and simplified for your understanding because I feel the standard medical illustration bores most people. Even if you don't pay any attention to these drawings, remember that the outermost, or surface, layer of your skin (epidermis) is made up of 10 to 20 fine layers of dead skin cells. We will go into simple, but extensive, detail about these cells that we call our basic skin.

In a very real sense, that's what this book is all about—getting down to basics. For without a proper understanding of the whys and wherefores of your skin and what to do for it, without the technique and procedure of practical application, it is only reasonable that you may be fearful of causing a makeup catastrophe on your own face.

UNFORTUNATELY, CONFUSION
REIGNS SUPREME

The various media give us such fragmented, out of context beauty information that we do not know how to utilize it. It is only natural to stay away from what is only half understood, although it is abundant and, in most instances, extremely useful information. But information is of no value until you know the underlying reasons, the why, when, and how to apply them to yourself. We are going to get it all together—first in our minds, and then in direct use upon our faces.

After a subject has been discussed in detail, you will find an "Action Capsule" at the end of the discussion to put it all together for you. This is a condensed, step-by-step review of the preceding information for easy reference. In the case of makeup which covers a group of subjects, there are three different "Action Capsules" at the end of the discussion of all the makeup products to put it all together for you. One is a complete daytime makeup, the second is a quick getaway makeup, and the third is an evening and gala makeup. By setting up the book on your dressing table or wherever you make up, you can use its guidelines before your own mirror with efficiency and expertise.

COMMUNICATIONS ARE IMPORTANT

Because I wish to avoid a lack of communication between you and me, it is very important to make sure that we agree about the meaning of several very commonly used words in cosmetic language. I find that even the most erudite women misuse some of these terms so let's get them cleared up at the outset.

You will notice that I never use the word *rub* (except when I say *"don't rub"*). I very often use the word *wipe*, even calling it to your attention by capitalizing it. There is definite reason for this. The wrong motions used daily on the face not only contribute to but accelerate the aging process. We're all (hopefully) going to grow old anyway, but who wants to get there ahead of time?

The word WIPE in cosmetic language means to remove any cosmetic with a sweeping, light, ONE-WAY, soft stroke. The word *rub* is not cosmetic language. It indicates the action of moving or rotating over the skin surface with pressure and friction in a back and forth motion. (Where the face is concerned, the word "rub" should be abolished!)

Here are some other cosmetic language terms:

Apply	To put, place, or spread on, using a gentle touch.
Blend	To spread smoothly to a sheer consistency or a thin, even layer using the pads of the fingertips or a sponge.
Circular Motion	To move gently or rotate in a circle or in a round pattern.
Dab	A quick, gentle tap or pat with a soft substance.
Dabbing	An on-and-off or in-and-out gentle tapping or patting.
Draw	To move or trace lightly in a particular direction.
Dust or Fluff	To apply a feather-whiff of a substance (usually powder) lightly over the skin.
Press	To exert a slight pressure, gently.
Spread	To apply, extend, or distribute evenly in a thin layer.
Stroke	To softly pass the hand across in one direction.
Sweep	A steady continuous stroke or movement.
Taut	To hold gently in one place, only slightly extending the skin.

In addition to *rub,* the other big no-no is:

Stretch or Pull	To expand or extend in length from one point to another; to draw tight or taut; to strain or enlarge by tension.

I do not wish to imply that your face is as fragile as that of a china doll, but it is most certainly not a football to be kicked around. And believe it or not, many women do just about that. Moderation is the keynote and gentleness the maxim.

WHY ALL THE CONFUSION?

As I said before, there are no villains, but responsibility must be squarely faced. All of us are individually innocent but collectively we have contributed to your present confusion. Buck-passing and reproaching others are among the oldest games in any business where there are related components that comprise a whole industry.

Added to this, many dermatologists contradict one another in print as well as in their offices on almost any superficial skin or cosmetic subject. The *real* problems are not in such dispute. Some dermatologists will readily admit that they do not want to be considered glorified cosmeticians. And well they shouldn't, for they are doctors who are vital for real skin disorders such as acne or psoriasis. Many accuse the cosmetic laboratories of fraudulent and worthless products and in *some* cases, with good reason.

The cosmetic chemists accuse the marketing and advertising people in their own companies of making overzealous claims for the products they develop in the laboratory. But sometimes they too can be overzealous about the theory and concept of a formula and therefore the resulting benefits of the product advertised to the consumer. Yet, I see and hear of a new integrity trying to break through.

The marketing and advertising people create the glorified product information (in this I, too, have been guilty). Creativity leads to fantastic claims for some products, for competition among cosmetic companies is very keen. The marketing, advertising and public relations people pass the information along, with potential sales in mind, to women's magazines and other media. These, in turn, interpret the information into the written and spoken word, portraying a glamorous but often confusing, and sometimes totally misleading, concept.

The editors are responsible to their publishers. The publisher is economically dependent on the advertiser, who is the company that started this round robin in the first place. And on it goes . . .

Everyone professes his or her own honesty and integrity, and appears to be sincere. And it is not hard to believe your own rhetoric when you are caught up in the swim of things. Who then should we believe? The answer is to listen to the voice of our own good common sense (which I believe most women possess). Listen to all and take what seems to be reasonable from a few—by knowing your basics.

PART I
YOU AND
YOUR SKIN

Your Skin

All women are beautiful—no matter what their age. But they could be more beautiful and, of course, some more beautiful than others. The idea is to look one's most beautiful at any age and this is something every woman alive can easily achieve.

With knowledge and a little determination, there are so many women who could be lovelier than they are. Most have good skin that could and should be better, skin that could be alive with radiance and bloom. Skin has to maintain a level of conditioning to keep its naturalness. To assume it is automatically possessed of this or that characteristic with doing little or nothing, leads to skin disaster.

Disregard and lack of caring has never been synonymous with natural, nor will it ever be! With improper care, often due to ignorance, many women do not appear as clean, fresh, or vibrant as they might. The health of their skin is in double jeopardy from lack of care and lack of protection. Doing little or nothing to and for your face is not allied to the current casual look in clothes. By the same token, hoping extravagant makeup will personify youth and glamour is also a mistaken notion.

Are you one of these women? Have you heard words to this effect before somewhere? Words like these, no matter how often they are heard, just do not seem to sink into these women's consciousnesses. The words do not seem to make a lasting impression. If you are one of these women it is my utmost, honest, and sincere intention to get through to you—to make you finally do something for yourself. If only a minimal but correct routine is undertaken, you will be one thousand percent better for it.

Now, let's talk about health. While the health of one's skin is

13

very much dependent on external care, internal care plays a vital and significant role. Good eating habits, which simply means well-balanced meals and vitamin supplements, lots of water to drink, regular elimination, proper rest, and exercise all contribute to glowing, beautiful skin. Worry, stress, and aggravation will take its toll. In short, overindulgence or deficiencies of *any* kind will cause aging in addition to being deleterious to one's health. Need I say more?

I have addressed myself to those over the age of 30 (and those approaching it) for several reasons: You share more common problems than younger age groups which permits me to be more effective. You have arrived at an age that is sometimes psychologically unsettling. When one hits 40, it can be emotionally devastating and only another 40-year-old woman knows how you feel. The 50s present a challenge to your cosmetic approach requiring a reappraisal and new techniques to compensate for sagging features. But there is a brighter side—the attention and care you had to lavish on others during your twenties has somewhat subsided and you now have more time to devote to Number 1, yourself!

Your appearance is important! It is not only important to you but to those you love. I've heard many a flip remark by women who say they "simply can't be bothered," when in reality they don't know what to bother about.

MAKEUP? ANYTHING IS EASY WHEN YOU KNOW HOW!

Know-how is the answer! There is no magic to applying makeup. The trick is simply know-how and the know-how is really simple. We call it "technique." And all it requires is knowing the proper fundamentals!

If you don't understand the many products and colors available to you, you are not alone. Many women are overwhelmed by the vastness and variety of it all. Makeup fashions always seem to be changing and although you might like to incorporate the latest trend in your personal routine, perhaps the technique seems too complicated because it has not been spelled out—it's begging for further interpretation. A common complaint from women sounds like this, "I read that article, you know, the one that said 'experiment.' Well, I followed the directions and you should have seen me—I looked so overly made-up. I don't know what was wrong, the instructions or me. I think I need something more personalized—more clearly defined—telling me exactly what to do and where to stop." If you also experimented, perhaps you didn't feel clean, or the result was inconsistent with your own personality—the way you view yourself.

Do experiment with the various individualized ideas in this book to arrive at a more natural look for you, and then you will be in a position to adapt new ideas as they come along. But do so only if you wish. If you are content with a natural look you have mastered (that's not a cliché, a lovely, natural appearance does take mastering), then stay with it. Fads and fashions come and go and there is no need to feel you must use every new trick that arrives on the scene. And well you shouldn't! The aura of glamour in print and commercials is just too much for many women. It doesn't take into consideration a certain practicality in terms of the individual. Still, it is wise to keep an open mind because no one wants to be behind the times.

WHAT IS A GOOD MAKEUP?

A good makeup is one that looks beautiful on *you,* regardless of brand or price; one that is easy and quick to apply; one that will last from morning till evening with only minor repair; one that looks continuously fresh and clean; one that looks and feels natural! All brands of color cosmetics fulfill these prerequisites *if* you know how to use them in combination. You will . . . before you finish this book.

Makeup is good for your skin. Make no mistake about that! You will have a far lovelier complexion for the rest of your life if you use makeup on a day-to-day basis than if you use nothing at all. It is a misleading idea that your skin has to continuously breathe free. Incidentally, the skin does not breathe for it does not take in oxygen from the air. (Oxygen is supplied from the lungs, then is carried to the skin by the blood vessels.) Naturally, the skin should rest. A healthy balance in everything is necessary for normality. A resting or recuperating period is necessary at night for you, as well as for your complexion.

On a day-to-day basis, makeup benefits your skin by protecting it from the elements, sudden temperature changes, pollution, wind, reflected glare, and especially from the sun (more about that later). Makeup constantly lubricates your skin by reinforcing your moisturizer. (And, much more about that later too.) These are two most important factors for skin maintenance and a healthy looking complexion.

A DRESSING TABLE?

A dressing table does not have to be the stereotype of one as such. It can be almost anything: a bedroom desk, a shelf in your bathroom, even the tank top of the toilet. The dressing table is anywhere that you have all your cosmetic preparations and makeup assembled. They should be organized in one place for your convenience and efficiency. Almost nothing is more frustrating than having to hop from one place to another in the midst of your morning or evening routine to pick up this or that.

If you haven't got it all together, why not make a mental note to do so now. And when you do get to it, why not weed out the collection of old, unused heavy lipsticks, foundations, rouges—those products you've probably been saving for years—they provide only clutter. The newer ones, and I'm sure you already own most of them, have a lighter, sheerer composition that is more in keeping with today's natural look.

To help get things organized, I suggest plastic trays with compartments to keep small items easily accessible. They are available in all price ranges.

TRULY ESSENTIAL BEAUTY TOOLS
Magnifying Mirrors

Billions of dollars are spent each year on toiletries. With all the cosmetic products women buy, and all their accumulated knowledge, *neglect* of their faces is widespread. The reason is simple—they cannot see!

One of the most essential cosmetic aids you can own is a lighted, magnifying mirror, especially for seeing the quality and state of your skin maintenance. It is really an indispensable health and beauty tool; you cannot care for small blemishes if you cannot see them distinctly. I know many of you will say, "Oh, I can't stand to look at myself in one of those mirrors. I don't want to see!"

Well now, let's be perfectly frank. If you can't be honest with yourself, who in this world can you be honest with? Better than anyone else, you know yourself! Take a good look to see if you are mismanaging your skin care. If so, I guarantee the mirror will reward and provide you with greater convenience and skill in the application of all your cosmetics.

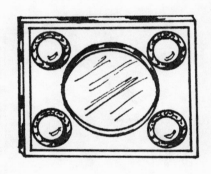

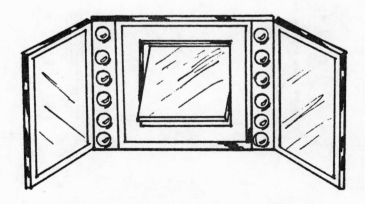

There are many models to be had
between these two versions. . . .

For those countless women who use their bathroom mirror and sink as their dressing table, there is a very easy, convenient, and inexpensive way to convert them into more efficient makeup centers. Bathrooms are notorious for bad overhead lighting, and good lighting is the first prerequisite to good skin care and makeup application. A mirror should be surrounded by light—a single overhead fixture is wholly inadequate. Strips of lights (see drawing) can be purchased at any electrical supply house or lighting and lamp store and can be installed on either side of your medicine chest. You can then add a magnifying mirror which permanently sticks to the mirror door by means of its own adhesive. These small additions can make a world of difference in your bathroom.

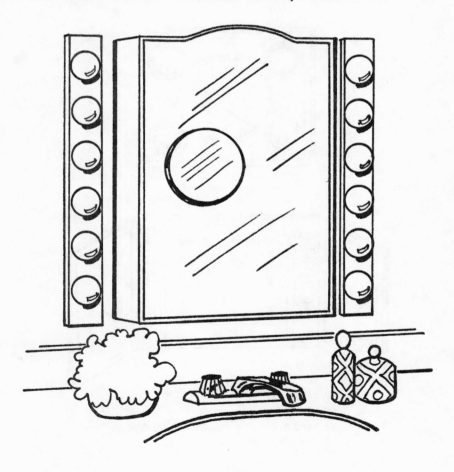

Beauty Tools for Your Dressing Table

ESSENTIAL
Tissues
Cotton balls or pads
Cotton swabs
Free-standing magnifying mirror
Hand mirror
Brush and comb
Eyebrow brush
Eyeliner brush (fine, thin sable bristles)
Lipstick brush, crayon, or pencil
Tweezers
Damp sponge or hand towel (used to wipe fingertips between
    applications of makeup, but not necessary if wash basin is
    readily accessible)
Wastepaper basket

NOT ESSENTIAL, BUT WORTH CONSIDERING
Cosmetic sponges
Small, soft complexion brush
Soft, sable powder brush
Terry cloth head band
Makeup cape to protect clothing
Small scissors
Eyelash curler

Undoubtedly, there are other beauty essentials that you would
like to incorporate on your dressing table if space permits, such as
perfume, nail enamel, hand and body lotion, etc. But since this
book deals with the face, I have listed only those items essential
to it.

Cosmetic Preparations and Makeup

ESSENTIAL
Night cream
Cleansing cream or lotion
Soap, properly suited to your skin
Skin freshener or astringent

Complete moisturizer (to be used when not wearing
    makeup)
Under-makeup moisturizer
Tinted foundation (base)
Under eye concealer or highlighter
Blusher (rouge in any form)
Powdered blusher (for touch up)
Loose face powder and puffs
Eyebrow pencil (if needed)
Eyeshadow
Eyeliner
Mascara
Lipstick

NOT ESSENTIAL, BUT WORTH CONSIDERING
Lip gloss
All-in-one tinted foundation and powder in compact (used
    when not wearing a complete makeup)
False eyelashes and glue
Special throat cream
Special eye cream

Your Handbag

To organize your essential take-along makeup, I suggest a small, zippered, fabric cosmetic bag, so that you do not have to probe around the bottom of your handbag when you want something. A suggested list would contain:

Lipstick and Lipbrush
Compact containing translucent powder
Compact powdered blusher
Automatic mascara and eyeliner
Eyeshadow

At Your Place of Business

For your office drawer or locker you might like to duplicate the makeup list in small convenient sizes. Many of these are packaged in plastic containers which makes them handy to take with you when you travel.

Your
Skin Structure
(It's Important to Know!)

This simplified illustration is greatly magnified to show just one hair follicle. Actually, there are 95 to 100 oil glands and 650 sweat glands per square inch of skin. The output of water is several hundred times greater than that of oil.

Your skin is divided into three distinct sections, each being a main layer:

The outermost layer is the *epidermis (stratum corneum)*. It consists of anywhere from 10 to 20 layers of dead skin cells. These cells adhere to one another tightly, except for those nearest the surface where they are continuously shed. The total thickness could well be represented by the page in front of you. As you turn the page, take note of its thickness. Two pages approximate the depth of 20 layers. For something so thin and compressed, it is sometimes hard to believe that our skin is so durable.

Below these 10 to 20 layers, is a barrier layer *(stratum lucidum)*. This is not a main layer but is part of the epidermis. The barrier layer is not a clearly defined structure, but it resembles a thin membrane. It acts as a regulator for what can be absorbed from the skin's surface, as well as for the loss of fluids from the body. The barrier layer can only be penetrated by a few specific cosmetic ingredients, and by more numerous medical ingredients, as well as toxic ingredients. This is why anything other than cosmetically formulated products or medically approved topical applications should not be applied to your skin. The skin, partic-

21

ularly in the eye area just below the eyes is exceedingly thin. Along with the eyelids it is the thinnest skin of your entire body.

The *epidermis* and *dermis* are firmly cemented together to form one membrane. The *dermis* is the true living skin. Immediately beneath these two main layers is the subcutaneous fat tissue containing a network of arteries and branches that supply blood and tissue fluids to the *dermis*. The lower portion of the *dermis* is merged with *collagen* and *elastic fibers* to give the skin strength and elasticity and the capacity to stretch and bounce back. The *dermis* also houses nerve fibers, blood vessels, connective tissue, hair follicles, oil and sweat glands.

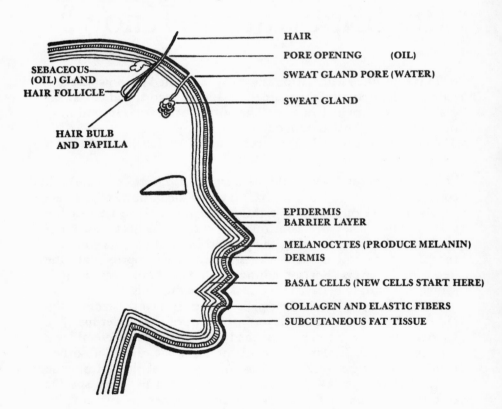

HAIR

PORE OPENING   (OIL)

SWEAT GLAND PORE (WATER)

SWEAT GLAND

SEBACEOUS (OIL) GLAND

HAIR FOLLICLE

HAIR BULB AND PAPILLA

EPIDERMIS
BARRIER LAYER

MELANOCYTES (PRODUCE MELANIN)
DERMIS

BASAL CELLS (NEW CELLS START HERE)

COLLAGEN AND ELASTIC FIBERS
SUBCUTANEOUS FAT TISSUE

The *sebaceous* (oil) glands are more abundant in the nose, cheeks, forehead and chin areas than any other part of the body. *Sebum* (oil) is a complex of salts, acid oils, water and waste products from the blood.

Just below the barrier layer there are new live cells constantly reproducing and pushing up toward the skin's surface to eventually die. Your skin is forever renewing itself from the live cells that travel toward the surface to become what is known as *keratin,* the exposed, dead, flattened cells we call our skin—the outermost layer of the epidermis. The complete renewing cycle takes anywhere from 15 to 20 days. The invisible shedding of dead skin cells goes on 24 hours a day. The greatest activity probably occurring while you sleep.

This is why you can have a clearer and healthier, virtually renewed skin in three weeks time! And, it could be a far more lovely, glowing skin that you now own. All it takes to reprogram your skin are the correct cleansing and lubricating procedures along with good health habits.

YOUR NATURAL PROTECTION

The *sebaceous* glands secrete oil (*sebum*) via a short duct into the necks of the hair follicles. Obviously, not all hair follicles produce hair, otherwise we would have hair all over our faces. The opening of the hair follicle in the skin thus becomes a pore, and you know what pores are!

The *sebum* is a highly complex mixture of fats. It travels upward through the hair follicle and penetrates it and the surrounding layers of skin to take part in forming a greasy film on the skin surface known as the *acid mantle.*

Simultaneously, the sweat glands are constantly releasing water. Each gland has its own pore to excrete sweat, this type of sweat produces no odor. The sweat is actually water which is imperceptible on the skin (you are unaware of it because you do not see or feel it). So you see, you actually have two different types of pores on your face, the *sweat pore* being the smaller of the two, but far more numerous. The water and oil mix together to form an emlusion, which is a coating or thin film over the entire face. This is

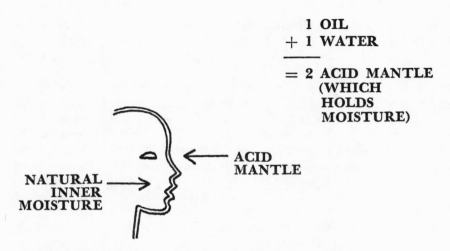

1 OIL
+ 1 WATER
─────
= 2 ACID MANTLE
(WHICH
HOLDS
MOISTURE)

←─── ACID MANTLE

NATURAL ──→ INNER MOISTURE

actually the *acid mantle,* which helps maintain a normal pliability of the skin by curbing the loss of water that is constantly being supplied from within. In everyday language, we call this moisture.

The *sebaceous* oil glands lie close to the hair follicles which provide the housing for each hair shaft. The follicle is the passageway to the pore for both hair and oil *(sebum)* .

When all is functioning normally, this "pipeline" is a one-way street leading to the surface of your skin.

When all is not functioning well, that street becomes blocked at the end—in the pores. Backing up on a one-way street is not only against manmade law, it is against the law of skin structure and the "traffic fine" is in blackheads, whiteheads, pimples, cysts, and worse.

Unfortunately, we are forced to remove much of the natural *acid mantle* in order to keep our skin clean and healthy. Fortunately, however, the body has the natural capacity to quickly replenish this vital film. But its quickness and capacity is also dependent upon you. This is where moisturizing fits in. So you see, a moisturizer is not only a cosmetic but a health preparation.

When you do not cleanse thoroughly, thinking you might be stripping away the natural *acid mantle,* dirt and bacteria of all types will attack the pore openings, clogging and backing up the natural flow of oil. A blackhead is a plugged up *sebaceous* (oil) gland. You may appear to have blackheads due to clogged up pores from the environment.

THE EFFECTS OF THE
SUN ON YOUR SKIN STRUCTURE

Pigment producing cells are called *melanocytes*. They produce *melanin*, tiny granules dispersed in the bottom layers of the *epidermis*, which accounts for your skin color—black, brown, yellow, white. There are about 60,000 *melanocyte* cells per square inch of skin.

Sunlight stimulates the *melanocytes* to produce more pigment. This increase results in darkening skin—a suntan, or worse, a sunburn. When you stay out of the sun, the excess pigment is gradually lost in the natural shedding process, and so your tan sheds too. It is true that the darker the *natural* skin, the less it will suffer skin damage over the years. But, oh that damage!

The sun's ultraviolet rays are terribly and irreversibly damaging and aging to your skin. This is a fact that has been known for many, many years by doctors and other knowledgeable people. But only now do you hear and read more about it.

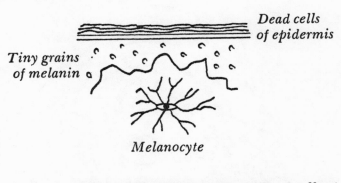

Melanocyte

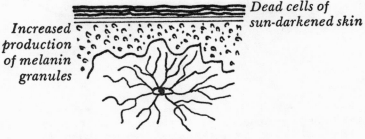

Stimulated Melanocyte

Still, however, many try to justify their sunning on the basis that it gives them a healthy appearance. It is not healthy! They simply like the tanned look it temporarily gives them. What do you do with people who won't listen? (I'm one of them in another area. I won't give up smoking*.) The only common-sense thing to do is preach moderation, and show them there is a way to circumvent the situation, at least partially.

Have your fun in the sun—summer or winter; north, south, east or west. Enjoy your sports—swimming, skiing, tennis, golf—but use protective outer clothing at every possible opportunity. Always wear a big hat when not actively engaged in a sport, and a smaller one with a sun visor when you are. Wear sunglasses with a good protective lens to help you avoid squinting (the more you squint, the more it imbeds those tiny laugh lines). Sit under large umbrellas which cut the ultraviolet rays by 50 percent. Use makeup

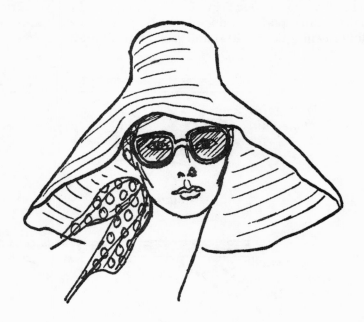

---

* Contrary to popular belief, smoking does not prematurely age or wrinkle skin according to the latest research reports. But of course this does not negate its known hazards to your health.

and most important of all, take along that tube or bottle of sunscreen. A product containing the ingredient *PABA* is the most effective sunscreen developed to date, and a really good sunblock contains 5 percent PABA—look for it on labels when you buy. Labels also indicate a protection factor (PF) on a scale of 1 to 10. One that blocks out most of the sun's ultraviolet rays will be in the range of 8 to 10 (logically suited to the face and neck if not the entire body). Even more important than taking the tube or bottle of sunscreen/sunblock along is to *use* it. Continually use it, and then think about using it some more. In other words, be conscious, *very conscious,* of the sun! Imagine you are in an enclosed 20-square-foot cancer-producing laboratory and you have to shield your face and body to keep cancerous rays off and away from you.

The other important thing to remember is to never, never deliberately seek the sun when it is unnecessary. By that I mean sun-

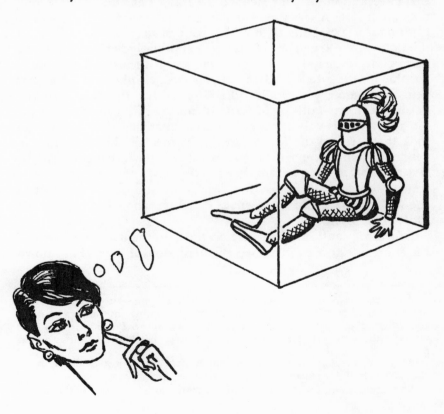

bathing, lying in the sun for the express purpose of tanning, unless you are of Types C or D of the following complexion types:

Type A　　Your skin burns but does not tan—usually very fair women.

Type B　　Your skin burns and tans lightly—fair to medium complexions.

Type C　　Your skin burns less and more readily tans—usually medium to olive complexion types.

Type D　　Your skin tans but does not burn—you're just plain lucky!

Be honest with yourself when you classify your skin type. You're fooling no one but yourself if you can't honestly say your skin type fits into the latter two categories. Even then, your face may not be able to take the punishment that your body* can withstand, and extra precaution for your face is a necessity. Let's face it, how long does a tan last? A week or two at the most? What you are accomplishing is to permanently burn up your protein *collagen* fibers in the *dermis*, the true skin. This has a cumulative effect. Each and every time you expose yourself to the sun it records another deep wrinkle for the future.** The result is aged, wrinkled, and leathery skin long before you would otherwise acquire the deep wrinkles of old age, to say nothing of actually causing skin cancer. Even the old-age wrinkles will be more accentuated at that time, if you can look that far into the future. In this regard, the hardest thing to get across to our teenage daughters (sons, too) is that the cumulative effect starts even before they are teenagers,*** and they could conceivably look 45 before they reach 30 if they continually sit in the sun. (I know. I have a teenage daughter who still gives me *the look:* "Oh, Mom!")

One more caution: If you are on the Pill, the ultraviolet rays of the sun can cause an increased pigmentation of your skin known

---

* You may want to use a sunscreen in the PF range of 4 to 6 on your body to permit it to tan. It would seem we are wisely coming into an era of using two different preparations at the same time. However, I think a truly wise woman will use the (PF) 8 to 10 sunblock all over her body as well as on her face.

** A sunlamp has the same detrimental effect and is just as damaging as the sun's rays, if not more so, because of its close proximity.

*** Limited doses of sun for teenagers with active acne can be beneficial.

as *photosensitivity*. (This same reaction can occur with antibacterial soaps, medicated cosmetics, perfumes, antiseptic creams, and hair conditioners.) This appears as mottled and darkened areas of the face and body. Again, a good sunblock is essential, particularly on areas given to discoloration. If mottling should appear, see a dermatologist.

There are some tanning processes that won't damage the skin and can be used by those who must have a tanned look. They are cosmetic bronzers and chemical indoor tanners and are perfectly safe if you test first to make sure that you have no allergic reaction. (See page 124 for patch test.)

PREVENTIVE CARE
MEANS PROTECTION—PROTECTION
MEANS PREVENTIVE CARE

This is important to both the outer and inner layers (*epidermis* and *dermis*) of your skin.

If the inner layer is damaged, it cannot replace itself. There is no way to repair it other than cosmetic surgery. (Also, a face lift cannot alter the quality of the epidermis, only its contour placement.) The *collagen* and *elastic fibers* located at the underside of the dermis control the skin's elasticity and are responsible for the skin's tone. The flexibility it provides allows the various motions we all make as we talk, eat, smile, laugh, yawn, squint, pout, grimace, wrinkle our brows, and so on. The collagen and elastic fibers can stretch and bounce back with all these motions but, with time, they begin to get weary and less flexible. They become more solid, and that is when skin begins to sag.

Naturally, one has to use facial expressions, or be robbed of the joys of life. But bad facial habits are not necessary to display one's emotions. Mannerisms that could be avoided, such as constantly cupping one's chin or cheek in the hand, will take their toll and put more strain on the elastic fibers and accelerate the aging process.

By the same token, facial exercise and deep massage put a strain on the collagen and elastic fibers causing them to wear down and eventually to break. It is a misleading idea to think one can tone up or even prevent a sagging skin by firming up the facial muscles. One has very little to do with the other and such measures can actually cause damage. A knowledgeable woman deliberately avoids professional facials unless her face is treated tenderly by an operator who handles it with utmost caution and extreme gentleness.

Of course, the most damage to your skin's collagen results from constant exposure to the sun, which without a doubt plays a more important role in the physical aging of skin than the aging process itself. Even normal light takes its toll, and that is one reason why makeup is a great protection. Lipsticks and foundations which contain a sunscreen are that much more protection if one spends a lot of time outdoors.

While there are limitations to the extent that one can protect the collagen and elastic fibers within the skin's dermis, you are in complete control when it comes to the care of the outer layer of the skin, the epidermis, because you have physical access to it. With know-how you have the capability of maintaining and preserving its health and appearance, and unlike the collagen, the epidermis has its own intrinsic capacity to self-replace.

Skin Types: Are You Really Sure of Yours?

Many women have incorrectly diagnosed their skin type. It is extremely important that you classify your face accurately. Regardless of what skin type you had when you were younger, it has changed. And, it will continue to change, gradually becoming drier, but not necessarily *dry*.

More women think they have dry skin than the ones who actually possess it. More often it is a combination skin with oily areas and drier patches, and this type of skin must be treated as the combination it is. Only as we grow older—into our 50s, 60s and beyond—do we truly have dry skin. This is due to the slow down of the sebaceous (oil) glands and their output of oil (*sebum*) as well as evaporation of too much water from the skin cells. This is not to say every woman over the age of 50 automatically has a dry skin, nor is it to say, that a woman of 30 can't have a dry skin. But, remember a lot more women *think* they have dry skin that they actually do.

I suggest you read all the skin profiles. It is conceivable that you may have excessively oily skin, thinking you have dry skin. Make absolutely certain what your skin type is. If you have misdiagnosed yours in the past, you have been using the wrong methods and the wrong products. The right products, procedures, and techniques will make all the difference in the world between good skin and glorious skin!

31

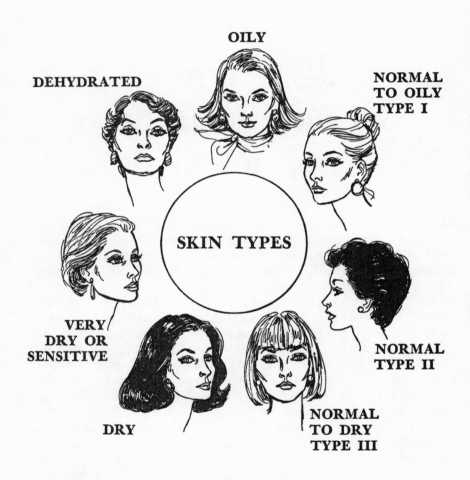

As time goes by . . . your skin may get drier—but not necessarily dry.

To typecast your skin, you must first cleanse very thoroughly. Use the Action Capsule on page 85 and then take a good long look in a strong light, preferably with a magnifying mirror.

Profile of an Oily Skin

The forehead, between eyebrows, nose, chin, cheeks and below cheekbones are *continuously* oily. You have enlarged pores due to dilation from too much oil. The skin texture appears coarse and you may have a slight redness or it may have a yellowish thin scaliness (some women think this is dry skin, but it is caked skin). You may have occasional or frequent skin eruptions; blackheads often occur. Oily skin is sometimes itchy and you may have dandruff. You may also have scaling or itching in the corners at the sides of your nose. The complexion tone is not quite clear, but when your face is completely cleansed, you have a shiny, glossy surface.

Profile of Normal Skin: Combination Types

Type I: Normal to Oily

Sides of face can range from normal to dry to quite dry. The greater portion of the T-zone—the center portion of the face—is oily. You may have a buildup of caked skin cells in the nose area and/or scattered blackheads or pimples on the forehead and

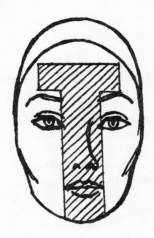

around the nose. Your T-zone has larger pores than the sides of your face. You may also have a thin yellowish scaliness in the central portion. In some women, this profile is exactly the reverse—although it is rare. The center portion of the face is normal and the sides are oily.

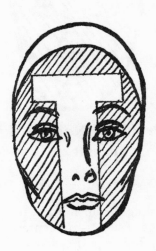

Type II: Normal

You have a fairly consistent (all over) not too oily, not too dry, skin. It is fine-textured with no visible pores and is smooth to the touch with a velvety, silky feel. It has a healthy glow and the surface appears to be translucent.

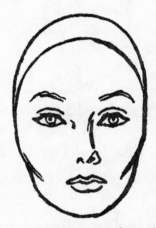

Type III: Normal to Dry

The major portion of your face is slightly dry or normal and generally fine textured. Your T-zone—the center portion of your face—is somewhat oily, perhaps on the nose and chin, or the oiliness may extend to the center of the forehead and between the eyebrows. You may have some laugh lines.

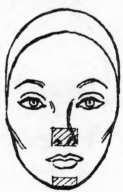

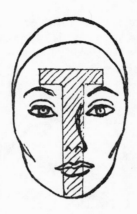

Profile of Dry Skin

Your face is dry in the central portion as well as dry to very dry at the sides. It often feels tight and uncomfortable. When your face is completely cleansed it appears to have no shine or gloss. It is sometimes flaky, itchy, and easily chaps or cracks in cold or windy weather. You have fine lines to deep wrinkles in the eye area. The texture of your skin is actually fine without visible pores, but it sometimes looks dull or thick and/or feels coarse. You may or may not have dandruff on your scalp.

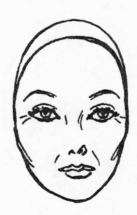

Profile of Very Dry, Sensitive, or Delicate Skin

You have all the signs of the above described profile for dry skin except that your fine textured skin is thin and often has a transparent look. It is easily irritated and reacts to internal and external changes as if from nervousness, for it may be pale and then suddenly flushed. It may or may not have red blotches in patches. Your skin requires special handling and special products that cater to your needs.

In addition, some women who bear all these signs also have oily patches, and this needs even further catering to. If your skin fits into this category, follow the instructions on page 80, using the suggested products, and *also* select a skin freshener from page 74 (Normal to Oily, milder fresheners). If the patches are extremely oily, select one of the stronger fresheners under the same heading. It is important to understand that these additional products be confined and used *only* on the oily patches. Avoid spreading your moisturizer onto these areas too.

Profile of Ultra-Dry Skin (Dehydrated)

You have all the characteristics of the profile for dry skin (see above), but in addition the moisture content of your skin is so low that it readily wrinkles. This may be due to an inherently dry skin that has become drier with advancing years and was not steadfastly cared for. In many cases it is from being a sun worshipper which over the years has also caused the skin to thicken. This woman may have a rich tan but it does not hide the fact that the skin looks shriveled and feels leathery.

There are other causes that will temporarily dehydrate the skin, such as excessive jet travel, being confined to overheated, low-humidity rooms, or simply not consuming enough liquids. Still other causes of dehydrated skin are certain medications, in which case you are undoubtedly in the care of a physician.

There are various degrees of dehydrated skin. If yours is seriously dehydrated, a physician or dermatologist should be consulted.

A Special Note to the Woman with Oily Skin

You differ from your sisters who have dry skin or normal skin only in the care you take and products you use. The basic technique remains the same.

Oily skin is healthy skin. It may provide an overall excess of oil, and it may be shielding against moisture evaporation naturally, but not necessarily. There are some women with oily skin where the water content is so low that the film on the face is almost pure *sebum*. These women should use a moisturizer with a high water content to provide the necessary moisture. These products are usually very thin and made mostly of water that is formulated with other ingredients to bond chemically more water. I realize this is often confusing to the woman with oily skin, but oil by itself is not moisture!

As years go by, oil production gradually decreases. You have probably already noticed that since the age of 25, the oiliness has diminished and it will continue to do so as you get older. Your consolation is that as you age, you will always be the woman with younger-looking skin than your contemporaries.

You need thorough cleansing, plus the additional use of an astringent that is specifically formulated for oily skin to help tighten pores and remove excess *sebum*. Resorcinol* is one of the ingredients to look for on labels, as it has a mild peeling action. Your cleansing program appears on pages 72–73. The use of clay masks at least once a week (more often is advisable) will deep-clean, drawing out excess oil, dirt, and cellular debris while it dries the skin. This type of mask has a mild abrasive action which polishes the skin, leaving it smoother and more even in texture. In addition to clay masks, do not overlook the use of exfoliants and saunas (see pages 86 and 88–89) . Your tinted foundation should be a water-in-oil or oil-free base. An oil-blotting gel used under your founda-

---

* Black women should avoid any product containing this ingredient as it might causes blotches.

tion is an excellent way to counteract an over-oily skin. It helps to retard shine and streaking. Use powder-based products, particularly blushers, but only over makeup. As I said before, you do not necessarily need a moisturizer, but it should be used if you notice any dry patches (particularly around the eyes). Remember too, that very few women with oily skin have throats and necks that are also oily, and a moisturizer may be needed in those areas.

Women who have *sensitive* oily skin must choose their products very carefully, particularly soaps (see page 72). It may be necessary to treat those sensitive areas as if you had a combination type skin, selecting skin fresheners and moisturizers from other skin type categories (pages 77–83) according to your particular sensitivity.

BLACK SKIN

There are at least 35 complexion shades among black women, but the skin types are essentially the same across races with only minor variations.

Refer to the various skin profiles (pages 33–38) and then check the profile for the black woman which follows for additional information and special cleansing instructions.

The care of black skin is as necessary as for any other complexion type and is no different in cleansing procedure or technique. It is just as important, if not more so, to remove all traces of soap with skin fresheners. Ashiness and, perhaps, itching are the prices you pay if this is not adhered to scrupulously.

There is also no difference in the aging process. But black women who care meticulously for their skin will look far younger, longer, due to the fact that the *melanin* is highly durable. The skin does not suffer as much from exposure to sun and light because the melanin screens out many of the harmful rays. This is not to say that you don't need protection from the sun. You also need a sunscreen even though your skin has a greater capacity to withstand the damaging rays of the sun.

These are special characteristics in addition to the profiles already outlined.

Oily Skin

See pages 33 and 72–73. For cleansing, use hot water (not burning hot) and one of the soaps especially formulated for oily skin outlined on page 72, or a medicated one. **Cuticura** or **Clearasil** are two good choices in this category. Even though astringents are indicated for oily skin, they are not recommended in your case. Instead use the milder skin fresheners outlined on pages 74–75 (Normal to Oily) or witch hazel.

Normal Skin

Combination Type I: Normal to Oily

This skin type is flexible and resilient. You need only proper cleansing to maintain healthier, clearer skin.

For cleansing use warm to hot water. **Ivory, Neutrogena Regular** or **Acne-Cleansing, Cuticura,** or **Clearasil** are soaps selected for your skin type. Use a mild skin freshener or witch hazel. Moisturize both face and neck avoiding the T-zone in the center portion of your face. **Jergen's Lotion, Vaseline Intensive Care,** and **Pond's Vanishing Cream** are several good choices.

Combination Type II: Normal

See page 35. Use the same products above or below. For a more comprehensive list of products, see pages 75–76.

Combination Type III: Normal to Dry

This skin may sometimes have an ashy tinge, a taut appearance, and it may have a shine, but the shine is not oiliness.

For cleansing use warm water and a mild soap such as **Ivory, Johnson & Johnson Baby Soap,** or **Basis.** Stay away from soaps containing perfume or detergents. Use a mild skin freshener—witch hazel is highly recommended. Moisturize your entire face and neck. **Jergens Lotion for Extra Dry Skin, Vaseline Intensive Care, Pond's Dry Skin Cream** and **Noxzema Raintree Moisture Maker for Normal to Dry Skin** are recommended.

Dry or Very Dry Skin

This is essentially the same as the profile on pages 36–37. In addition, your skin is tight, flaky, and sometimes fissured (with clefts or splits) . Chapping may also be a problem in cold weather.

For cleansing use lukewarm water and superfatted soaps. **Johnson & Johnson Baby Soap, Neutrogena Dry-Skin**, and **Dove** are but three good types for your skin. Use a very mild skin freshener. **Fashion Fair** and **Flori Roberts** are custom houses specializing in products for the black woman. Both have excellent skin fresheners for dry skin. Moisturize with any moisturizer formulated for especially dry skin. See pages 79–80.

A Special Note to the Black Woman

Black women are more prone to light and dark patches or blotches than whites. In order to avoid this pigmentation (color spots) , extra care must be exerted on your part.

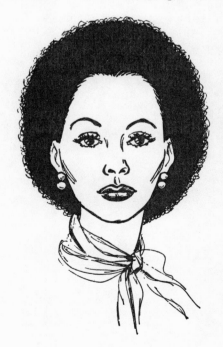

Trauma or undue shock to your face should be minimal or avoided altogether. While your skin has the ability to absorb more shock it is nonetheless more fragile than others. (See pages 88–89, Facial Saunas.)

With this in mind, blackheads, whiteheads, and pimples must be removed with extremely gentle pressure (see pages 97–99) in order not to bruise or damage the tissue. Bruises can result in permanent discoloration. Damage can result in *keloids* (thick growths of fibrous scar tissue). Even piercing one's ears at any age has all too often resulted in these unsightly growths, which can be treated by a dermatologist who injects medication causing the keloid to shrink. Or failing that, plastic surgery in some cases can sufficiently reduce or tend to eliminate the problem. (See pages 119–120.) For the same reason, you should avoid any form of exfoliation (skin abrasion), (see page 86). Saunas and masks are highly recommended.

If you have a prolonged pimple and you cannot remove it easily, see a dermatologist.

Cleansing Your Skin

#1, YOU

Your skin can be magnificently beautiful for most or even all of your life! The reason is that the deterioration of skin can be slowed down to a virtual standstill with proper care. I'm sure you've seen very old ladies, even in their 70s and 80s with beautiful skin, albeit they have the lines and wrinkles of old age. The

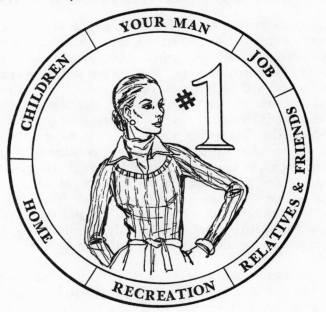

43

quality is there! Certainly heredity plays a part, but good genes without good maintenance does not insure healthy and lovely skin.

Sixteen, eighteen, or twenty-four hours of continuous *anything* on your face, without being thoroughly cleansed, is too much abuse for anyone's skin, regardless of type.

You might have been the average, young adult woman with many things to do and many things to worry about besides maintaining her skin. On some occasions, you might have been the girl who went to bed without having cleansed or removed her makeup. At 30, you become more knowledgeable, and realized it was high time to start thinking and paying attention to yourself. Taking care of Number 1 (need I remind you, it's *you*) is of prime importance, and there is absolutely nothing selfish or narcissistic about it. You have only one you! There is nothing better than to look and feel your best on every day—not just sometimes.

CLEANSING CREAM OR LOTION: WHAT IT IS, AND WHAT IT IS NOT!

A cleansing cream or lotion is a combination of emollients and detergents formulated to permit the easy removal of the greater portion of makeup, dirt, and grime. Actually, they belong in the category of *pre*cleansers, because they are not sufficient unto themselves for proper and correct cleansing. However, you will not find the word "precleanser" on the label of any cleansing product. The "pre" is omitted. You must know what a cleansing product is for, what it does, and what it does not do. It is not, by an stretch of the imagination, an adequate *total* cleansing procedure by itself.

This is where the most common and flagrant skin mistakes are made by countless thousands, perhaps millions, of women.

Women tissue off the cleansing product and think they are finished with the cleansing process. Some might go a step further and splash their faces with water. This is only slightly better, and still falls into the same destructive and disastrous skin cleansing category.

It really doesn't make very much difference which type of cleanser you use for it is only a preliminary step. It is not going to stay on your face long enough to do more than break down the dirt and grime, as well as the bulk of makeup. A cleansing cream or lotion does not take the place of soap and water for most all skin types.*

Moisture, Moisture, Everywhere! Confusing, Isn't It?

It is *impossible* to cleanse and leave a vitally necessary moisture film on the skin all in one application—and attain a "clean skin." Yet, many cleansing products offer both—cleansing and moisturizing—which leaves many women totally and utterly confused. Simply remember these are two entirely separate steps in your cleansing routine.

While the moisturizing ingredients of a cleansing cream or lotion help to soften the skin, it is of little consequence, for it is completely insufficient as far as performing as an actual moisturizer. This becomes obvious when you remember that a cleanser of any type must be completely removed, and all last traces again removed with a skin freshener or astringent for truly clean skin.

A cleansing cream or lotion or even baby oil may be used to cleanse your face initially. These precleansers are not soluble in water. There are products known as rinsable cleansers, which are similarly packaged and are water soluble, but they should not be confused with cleansing creams or lotions. Rinsable cleansers take the place of soap for those women who should not or will not use soap. Only in certain rare instances should a cleansing cream be considered a substitute for both preliminary cleansing with a cleansing cream or lotion, and the next step of washing with a rinsable cleanser or soap.

For removal of the day's makeup, dirt, and grime, you need a sufficient quantity of cleanser so that you will not drag or pull the skin with your fingers. It is important to use *upward* and *outward* light, stroking motions on your face, throat, and neck. DO NOT RUB. You may not be concerned with this practical idea now if you are hovering around 30, but take a long range view—be concerned with the future of your skin. All downward motions tend

---

* The exception is if you have very dry or sensitive skin that "hurts," or a dehydrated (ultra dry) skin. See pages 37–38 and recheck your skin type.

to pull the skin and make it sag downward. The cumulative effect is then compounded each and every time you apply a cream or cosmetic using the improper motions. Even when you use paper tissues, the same upward, outward motions should be used.

There has been some controversy recently over the use of paper tissues. You may have heard or read that you should not use tissues, because they leave a residue of wood fiber on your face.

CLEANSING MOTIONS

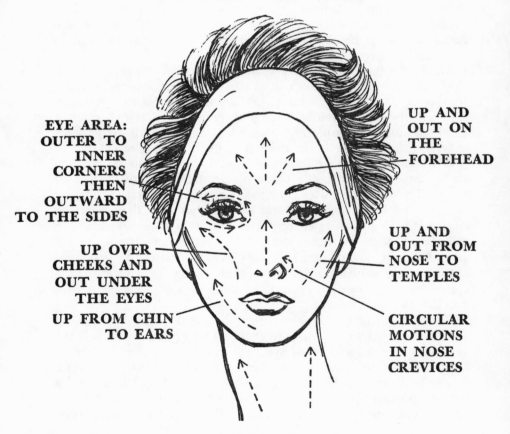

EYE AREA: OUTER TO INNER CORNERS THEN OUTWARD TO THE SIDES

UP AND OUT ON THE FOREHEAD

UP OVER CHEEKS AND OUT UNDER THE EYES

UP FROM CHIN TO EARS

UP AND OUT FROM NOSE TO TEMPLES

CIRCULAR MOTIONS IN NOSE CREVICES

Use the same motions for applying creams and lotions, tissuing-off, and using cotton saturated in skin freshener.

Whether they do or don't is unimportant and negligible. It would only have some significance if tissuing-off was the last thing you did in the cleansing process, and this is assuming the fiber scare was true in the first place. By now you know that tissuing off is one of the first steps in a proper cleansing procedure. Residue of any type is going to be completely removed. You want the skin on your face to last you, beautifully, for a lifetime!

SOAP AND WATER: WHERE, OH WHERE, HAVE YOU BEEN?

No matter what your age or skin type or what environment you live in, no matter what the climate or season of the year, proper cleansing every morning and night is absolutely vital to the health, well-being, and beauty of your skin.

The virtues of soap and water are many. Most skin types will thrive on them if given the chance and if the right soap is selected. Of all cleansing agents, soap should be your first choice. In most cases, it can be.

Most women who say they cannot use soap because it is too drying have probably made one of two mistakes and possibly both. They have previously used the wrong soap* for their complexions, or they did not properly rinse the soap off.

Soap is only drying to the skin if it is allowed to build up when a partial film is left on the face, and/or when a kind of soap not properly suited to the skin is used. The extra precaution of wiping away all last traces of residue with a skin freshener is part and parcel of any proper cleansing routine.

There are a few exceptions, namely a very dry, sensitive, or dehydrated skin. Women who have this type of skin—and they are usually older women (that doesn't mean 42 or even 52)—find it

---

* There are great differences in soap from one brand to another. Every soap is formulated with different ingredients and to different specifications. Some soaps are even patented. Take notice of your soap's outer wrapping. You might find a patent number on it. A patent is not obtainable from the U.S. Patent Office unless the new product is sufficiently different from that which already exists.

difficult to put practically anything on their faces. A woman whose skin easily chaps is also an exception. But most other women can and will greatly benefit from the use of a proper soap* expressly suited to their skin, *if they will only try!*

I have endeavored to place most of the well-known brands in their proper category by skin type so that you may select them more knowledgeably for your own particular skin type. It is not uncommon for a truly knowledgeable woman who can afford the very best, to have at her disposal two different types of soap. The one for her bath might be a popular deodorant soap or a fragrant French milled soap, while at her wash basin, you will most likely find a standard brand of commercial facial bar soap or a specialized imitation soap.

If it is possible to use true soap instead of detergent soap, then by all means do so. (An overall oily skin is an exception and may need a detergent soap.) If the effect of true soap seems to be too drying, then switch to another brand or to an unscented, mild, synthetic imitation soap, using plenty of clear rinsing water. It is not necessary to splash more than 20 times when you rinse. The time spent rinsing certainly should not exceed one minute. A total time of a minute and a half is more than sufficient for both soap and water. Use just enough water to remove the soap residue because *any* residue can become irritating. In any case, you will remove all last traces with your skin freshener regardless of what type soap you use. This important step cannot be omitted. Only in exceptional cases (the severely dehydrated skin) should this procedure be avoided. For this latter type of skin a dermatologist should be consulted.

The above mentioned skin type is the exception, rather than the rule, for most women are blessed with normal, healthy skin, even though it may range from very dry and sensitive to oily. However, I see women everywhere with dull-looking lifeless skin and it is needless, heartbreaking, and can easily be overcome. In healthy

---

* In today's society, women's buying habits put more emphasis on the color of soap (to coordinate with bathroom tile or towels) than on considering which soap is most beneficial to skin. This idea is ridiculous. Your skin is far more important than a perfectly coordinated bathroom (and I love a pretty bathroom). When the consumer starts demanding soap to correlate with her skin type, then more soap companies will manufacture and market their brands formulated for individual skin types in a variety of colors as well.

skin (which I remind you is the only type I am talking about) , the only time soap has a possibility of being irritating is when it is *left on the skin too long*. The only chance of being remotely drying is when it is not properly removed, and that means totally removed!

If, after reviewing the skin type profiles, you consider yourself very dry or ultra-dry (dehydrated), only then should you dispense with soap. Your alternative is a rinsable cleanser. This kind of product is used in place of all types of soap. You might consider it a replacement soap for it is soluble in water just as regular soap is.

Rinsable cleansers are also known as washable cleansing creams, milky cleansers, beauty milk baths. Make sure that the label on the product indicates "rinse with water" or "rinsable." These products are not to be confused with cleansing creams or lotions which are not water soluble. However, remember that rinsable cleansers are more difficult to remove with water because they do not lather as soap does. So extra rinsings with water and special care are necessary.

Interviewing Is the Name of the Game

Recently, I interviewed a typical woman as to how she cleansed her skin. Her answer went like this: "Well, I use soap and water on my face, sometimes." When I asked her, "Why sometimes?" expecting to receive the usual answer, "it's too drying for me," she surprised me by saying, "I use it sometimes because I usually get it in my eyes and I don't like that." Had this lovely lady been employing the proper cleansing procedure in the first place, such minor catastrophes would have been dealt with on the spot and her "sometime" distaste for soap and water would have been washed down the drain. Separate washing of the eyes with a soothing eyewash is the very next step.

Probably the most common complaint that crops up in my interviews with women who have previously used soap and water sounds like this: "But my face feels so taut after washing with soap." Here they usually make animated faces dropping their jaws into a stiffened position to demonstrate what I know can be a very uncomfortable feeling. I truly sympathize, but I also know that taut feeling is due to the wrong soap for the skin type. And even if a woman with dry skin should experience a slightly taut feeling, it is immediately alleviated when the correct after-procedure is put into practice. Your moisturizer, which is only two steps away, should be applied *within* the next minute—and believe me, you'll feel immediate relief. There simply is no excuse for that taut feeling. And as I will emphasize again and again the "correct cleansing procedure (which only takes three minutes) consistently used day-in and day-out is the difference between good skin and glorious skin." It is within your reach no matter how many birthdays you've seen since your 30th.*

Water Is the Original, Unique, and Natural Form of Moisture in or out of Your Skin!

There are women who complain that they don't like or cannot use water. This idea is almost laughable. It is pure myth! Water is the only commodity that truly softens skin. Nothing else has the same effect. Water is the ultimate moisturizer. Its only drawback is we cannot retain its moisture, for as anyone knows, water evaporates when exposed to air. (Think of clothes drying on a clothesline.) *This is one of the reasons we must use a moisturizer.*

Water temperature should always be tepid (lukewarm). Hot water, hot towels, *hot anything* can be damaging to the facial skin and you may intensify an already existing problem by continuing to use hot water if you do so now. The only exception to this is a woman who has an overall oily skin. For that matter, contrary to popular belief, cool or cold water has very little or no effect in closing the pores, although ice has some value.

Some women arrive at an age when they say, "water hurts my skin or makes it feel parched." Granted, this can happen, but it is for the most part a temporary discomfort. I find, usually, that this type of woman is already in the care of a physician or dermatologist, and of course, she should follow his advice. Far too many

---

* It is never too late! I've interviewed ladies well into their 60s who have beautiful "quality" skin. Upon probing the whys and wherefores, invariably it was due to their proper step-by-step maintenance regimens which they began in their late 40s or early 50s. These women openly admitted they had not taken correct care of their skin up until that time.

women have made this self-diagnosis for themselves to the detriment of their skin. All they really have to do is stay away from detergent type soaps—soaps with additives, deodorants, fragrance, even lemon. In cold weather, if you skin feels oversensitive, switch to a rinsable cleanser for a while and then go back to soap when weather conditions permit.

A morning cleansing routine is just as important as every night cleansing. It is a fallacy to think that morning cleansing is unimportant. Many women take the attitude, "I haven't been anywhere so how could I get dirty?" True, your skin is not *as* dirty as the night before, but it has been at its most active phase of shedding dead skin cells during the night, and it is important to remove this cellular buildup. You may omit the precleanser you would normally use to remove makeup, but use the rest of the regular cleansing routine.

For everyday washing, a clean, fresh washcloth is just abrasive enough for sluffing away dead surface cells. Also, a once-a-week cleanser in the form of a mask or abrasive exfoliator will keep your skin looking clear and fresh. More details will follow on these subjects later. (See pages 86, 87.)

Please, always observe the first law of facial hygiene. Only use absolutely clean equipment on your face. A washcloth should be a freshly laundered face cloth, not one previously used on any other part of the body. An abrasive cleansing sponge* of any type should be thoroughly rinsed out after using and should be your personal property alone. The same is true for complexion brushes.** Needless to say, always wash your hands before applying them to your face.

The only other alternative to cleansing, which completely eliminates the use of any water soluble product and water as well, is a deep pore cleansing cream or lotion. These products are used to remove makeup as well as the accumulation of dirt and grime. They are tissued off or removed with large wads of cotton. It takes several applications, especially if one wears makeup, to become even nearly clean. After using a deep pore cleanser, wipe your face

---

* Buf-Puf, from 3m Riker Laboratories is one of this type.

** Electrical or battery operated complexion brushes should be used only exerting *very* light pressure. Digging-in is not only unnecessary to attain the benefits, but potentially damaging to the skin's underlying structure.

thoroughly with cotton saturated in skin freshener to remove all last traces of the cleanser. Admittedly, it takes much longer and one uses a greater amount of the cleansing product, tissues, and cotton to complete the job. It is the third choice on the list of cleansing procedures and should be resorted to by women who feel they cannot use either of the preceding two methods.

Soap and Water Debate

It cannot be said too often: Proper cleansing is so vitally important to the health and appearance of your skin. And I find confusion and debate on this subject more than any other.

At this point, a very logical question on your part might be, "If I use a deep pore cleansing lotion or cream and a freshener to remove all traces of makeup, dirt, and grime, why do I even have to go near soap and water or rinsable cleansers?"

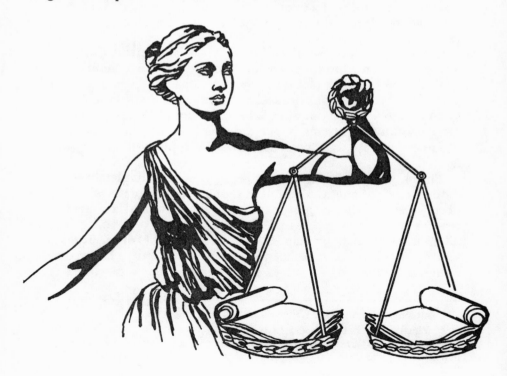

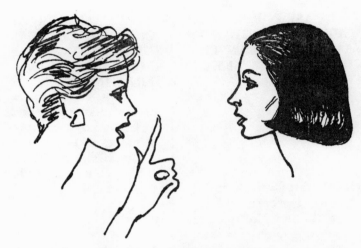

OK . . . Let's Debate It!
Soap and Water or Rinsable Cleanser Followed by Skin Freshener
vs.
Cleansing Cream or Lotion Followed by Skin Freshener

THE CASE FOR SOAP & WATER (INCLUDING RINSABLE CLEANSERS) FOLLOWED BY SKIN FRESHENER

I get rich lather and warm water dissolves the soap.

Well, my skin is sort of dry too, but I find soap and water creates more friction to remove caked matter and loosen blackheads. I like the speed; it's much faster.

THE CASE FOR CLEANSING CREAM OR LOTION FOLLOWED BY SKIN FRESHENER

I don't get lather with my cleansing cream. But I have dry skin and I think soaps are supposed to be drying.

THE CASE FOR SOAP & WATER (INCLUDING RINSABLE CLEANSERS) FOLLOWED BY SKIN FRESHENER

THE CASE FOR CLEANSING CREAM OR LOTION FOLLOWED BY SKIN FRESHENER

When I tissue off, I create friction too, and it removes caked matter and blackheads also, even though it takes me longer.

I think warm water is superior. I've been told it's the ultimate moisturizer. I know it softens my skin.

Well, cleansing creams soften, too.

Oh, but not to the same extent! Besides, I hear that warm water is "natural exercise" causing the blood vessels of the skin to dilate and later contract. And it feels so relaxing!

Is that a fact? Well, I have no answer for that one. But I do know that if you make a mistake and use water that is too hot, it may cause permanent thermal changes in your skin.

I know . . . so I use just enough soap and lukewarm water to remove the mass of creams, debris and makeup. And I even rinse with lukewarm water. You know it's an old wives' tale that cold

THE CASE FOR SOAP & WATER (INCLUDING RINSABLE CLEANSERS) FOLLOWED BY SKIN FRESHENER

water closes the pores. But I must admit cold water feels good sometimes.

Hm . . . let's see. That's almost 1800 years ago. I've heard from doctors that the medical value of soap has been recognized for 5000 years.

I don't have to pull and drag at my skin with tissues or cotton to remove most or all of my makeup and dirt, just enough to get the bulk of it. Soap and water washes the rest of it away.

THE CASE FOR CLEANSING CREAM OR LOTION FOLLOWED BY SKIN FRESHENER

I don't have to control the temperature of water. My cleansing cream melts at body temperature. And did you know that cold cream was developed in A.D. 200 by a Greek physician?

Well, cosmetic chemists haven't been at it that long, but they know what they are doing too.

It's true, I have to keep wiping and wiping in order to get practically all the makeup and dirt. Maybe sometimes I do pull and drag a little too much.

THE CASE FOR SOAP & WATER (INCLUDING RINSABLE CLEANSERS) FOLLOWED BY SKIN FRESHENER

It takes me one or two cotton balls to remove all the last traces of any residue with skin freshener.

Yes!

Cleansers of that type are not water soluble, so you are right back to a rinsable cleanser (or soap) again.

THE CASE FOR CLEANSING CREAM OR LOTION FOLLOWED BY SKIN FRESHENER

It takes me three to six cotton balls to remove all the last traces with skin freshener.

I guess I use more skin freshener too . . . and isn't it on my face for a longer period of time?

OK, I concede. How about if I use my deep pore cleanser and rinse my face with water, then apply my skin freshener?

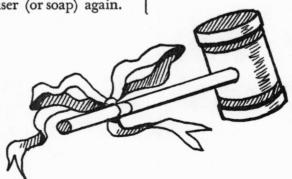

My case rests!
Just make sure you choose the right kind
of soap for your particular skin type!

YOUR PRECIOUS EYES
NEED SPECIAL ATTENTION, TOO!

Washing or flushing your eyes with an eye wash should be a regular daily care procedure and it fits very nicely into the cleansing routine.

Making up eyes that are anything less than clear and free of all debris is like putting makeup on a dirty face. You should cleanse your eyes before applying any makeup, moisturizer, or skin freshener.

After washing with soap and water and before using skin freshener (a freshener should never be used on the immediate area of the eyes), thoroughly saturate a cotton ball or pad with liquid eyewash and wipe the eyes from the inside to the outside corner. Using cotton is quicker and easier than using the eye cup usually supplied with this type of product. Use two pieces of cotton, one for each eye. Barnes-Hind's **Blinx,** Cooper Lab's **Dacriose,** Warner Lambert's **Ocurinse,** Wyeth's **Collyrium** are only four of the products of this type that you will find soothing, gentle, and refreshing.

Eye washes provide a marvelous wake-up feeling in the morning. At night, they remove all last traces of eye makeup after you have removed most of it with cleansing cream or special eye makeup removers. Using a ball of cotton saturated with cold water is also effective but doesn't quite have the soothing properties of the eye washes we are discussing. An eyewash is an isotonic solution and has the same pH balance as is normally found in eye tissue. Since products of this type should be kept in sterile condition, don't reuse a piece of cotton by reapplying it to the opening or neck of the bottle.

Eye drops, as opposed to eye wash, are usually (but not always) *vasoconstrictor* type products which "get the red out," such as Pfizer's **Visine** or Abbott's **Murine 2.** They are particularly helpful when applying makeup if any matter should form in the corners of the eyes. Squeeze a drop or two on a cotton swab and gently lift the debris from the corners. The excess moisture will run into the eyes giving immediate relief. And it will temporarily cause the blood vessels to contract, thereby eliminating red streaks, giving the eyes a clear, white, sparkling appearance. However, the blood vessels will later dilate of their own accord, usually within a few hours.

I am not particularly fond of using eye drops on an everyday basis. I think they have their place as an occasional pick-me-up,

but they are not a substitute for regular eye washing as part of
the cleansing procedure.

SKIN FRESHENERS:
YOU'RE A FUNNY ONE WITH
ALL YOUR NAMES!

For the purpose of clarity, the term freshener has been used to
cover the vast realm of this kind of toning product. These products vary mainly in the degree of alcohol strength, although their
basic purpose is the same—to balance, tone, clarify and cleanse
the skin, which makes it look smoother and firmer, and to give it
a cool, fresh feeling. Different names are used:

Astringents*	Refreshant lotions
Balancing lotions	Skin conditioners
Clarifying lotions	Skin fresheners
Exhilarating lotions	Skin tonics
Face washes	Toners**
Pore lotions	Toning lotions
Purifying lotions	Toning and refining lotions
Refinishing lotions	

Because of the lack of consistency from company to company,
these names often present a confusing picture to many women,
especially with respect to the amount of alcohol content each one
contains. The assistance of a beauty advisor or cosmetician is
needed to select the right freshener for you. This is just as important as choosing the right soap. It is not an item to be purchased
casually.

The use of a skin freshener is a vital and necessary part of the
cleansing procedure. The primary reason for using a freshener is to

---

* Astringent denotes that the product has a higher alcohol content than
others, and this should only be used by those women with oily skin.

** A toner usually contains ingredients to further help tighten the pores.
These ingredients are also present in astringents, but usually they are more
highly concentrated than in toners.

rid the skin *completely* of all other cleansing products used previously in the cleansing procedure, so that your skin is *super* clean. It contributes to the difference between good skin and glorious skin.

All these products, regardless of their names, contain alcohol as their active ingredient (unless the label indicates otherwise) in varying degrees of potency, astringent being the strongest of all. It is the alcohol content in these products that literally cuts through grease and traces of other matter left on your skin, even after you have splashed your face with water 30 or 40 times in the cleansing process. (Another reason why it is not necessary to spend so much time with water.)

Now, you may shudder at the thought of using alcohol on your face. The very word seems to scare many women for they immediately associate it with being terribly drying. But you should know that there are many kinds of alcohol, and it is a primary ingredient in many cosmetic formulations that you would never think of as drying. It is not of the strength with which you normally associate alcohol—usually 70 percent ethyl (rubbing type) alcohol. In all types of skin fresheners the specific alcohol has been diluted to be compatible with other pore tightening and circulation stimulating ingredients, such as *rubefacients* (*rube,* red; *facient,* that makes). Nevertheless, since it will remove every last trace of anything left on your face, it will simultaneously remove a portion of your natural moisture, the acid mantle, depending upon the strength of the individual skin freshener. This is one of the main reasons for using a moisturizer *immediately* after the freshener (but before it has completely dried). This almost total removal cannot be helped and it is not harmful when balanced with a supplementary moisturizer. It is actually very beneficial for it is the only method of getting to the basic skin to cleanse it of all foreign matter. Soap and water, even plenty of it, cannot do it alone.

While alcohol is a primary ingredient, the main ingredient in all skin fresheners is purified water (e.g., mineral water). Look at the label of any freshener and you'll see it is the first ingredient listed. (Even though some brands only list "water," still it must be purified.) Besides being essential to the formulation of the product, purified water serves a very definite purpose that you should be aware of: Tap water varies in different localities all over the country (and indeed all over the world)—some better, some worse, some hard, some soft. But more important, communities cannot rely on the absolute purity of their own water supply as harmful chemicals are becoming more and more prevalent. It is necessary not only to drink purified water, but to make sure that your washing water is purified for the final rinse, at least for your face and neck. Skin fresheners instantly and automatically provide this convenience. (Still another reason why 20 splashes of running tap water is adequate enough for rinsing.) Since the purified water in the freshener is the final water to touch your face it is advantageous to seal it in with your moisturizer.

A cotton ball or pad saturated with skin freshener is wiped all over the face and neck, even behind the ear lobes (but not on the eyes). The cotton will invariably show up somewhat dirty to downright dirty, even after you think you have washed thoroughly and rinsed with many splashes of clear water.

Please note: I said "WIPED." Do it gently, but firmly, using upward, outward motions. Patting, splashing, or dabbing will not accomplish the same purpose and the primary reason for using the freshener or astringent is defeated. Your skin is clean when all residues are completely wiped away. It may take one, two, or more saturated cotton balls to accomplish this, but keep going until the last cotton ball looks completely clean. Leave your face slightly damp—it will only take moments for the alcohol to evaporate. You are now ready to apply your moisturizer and you should do this posthaste. It will not only externally moisturize and seal in the purified water of the freshener, but it will also immediately allow your own natural moisture to replenish itself from within. Therefore, any drying effect from the alcohol is totally counteracted. You will not only look clean, you will feel clean and soft—and you know that's a great feeling!

There is a mistaken notion that skin fresheners will close the pores of the skin. While they do have a temporary constricting effect on the pores, they do not literally close them; they do aid in the improved appearance of the pores. But, what is more important, the right freshener chosen for the skin type balances the skin, especially in the case of combination types, where two fresheners of different strengths are needed for optimum balance and noteworthy results.

MOISTURE . . . MOISTURIZERS . . . AND MOISTURIZING

If you apply only one beauty rule, it should be to moisturize your face, throat, and neck at *all times*. If this book creates no other impression on you, *please,* let it be this one!

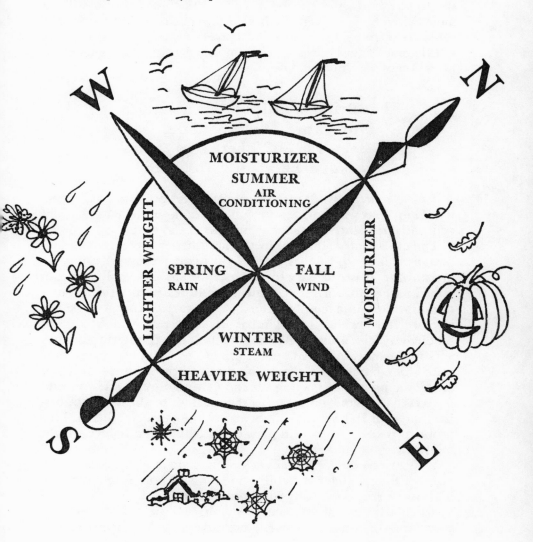

A moisturizer should be used regardless of the hour, locale, season, or climate—even in summer when hot weather naturally produces more oil (*sebum*). The trick here is to switch to a lighter weight moisturizer than the one you normally wear. Air conditioning and other external hazards make this a necessity. The only possible exception to this rule is if you have a very oily skin but, even in these cases, the neck and throat should still be moisturized because everyone has far fewer sebaceous oil glands in those areas. In cold winter months, every woman should use just a little more of her normal weight moisturizer, again paying extra attention to the throat and neck.

The Primary Purpose of a Moisturizer Is to Form an External Film . . . To "Sit" There . . . Not to be Totally Absorbed

Today, practically all modern moisturizers act in a dual capacity. They hold your own natural moisture in and chemically add additional moisture by means of emollients and water.

The emollients contained in the moisturizer are extremely important, but are to be considered a secondary reason for using the moisturizer. It is necessary to understand that the emollients contained in the moisturizer are quickly absorbed into the skin, but a thin film is simultaneously formed on the surface and must be left in place. This protection is vital and is the reason you should *not* blot it away with a tissue. Blotting is absolutely counterproductive.

Give the moisturizer an opportunity to set before applying your tinted foundation. (This is a good time to brush your teeth if you are in the process of making up and getting dressed.) If you find it necessary to blot, you are using too much or too heavy a moisturizer, and your skin simply cannot absorb the extra emollients. This problem is resolved by using less or switching to a lighter weight moisturizer.

Moisturizers do not contain heavy pigments (color) because the pores of the skin have the ability to grab and hold color particles. This is the reason why any color product such as blusher or rouge (particularly, powdered rouge) should not be put directly on your skin. They are occlusive (pore clogging). A moisturizer will not clog the pores unless you use one designed for an altogether different skin type than your own.

A moisturizer alone must be a completely separate product, not in combination with any other product or application. Alone, it forms an invisible screen with still other benefits:

- It acts as a barrier or shield against all outside environmental elements including sun, wind, and pollution.
- It lubricates to make the skin feel soft, silky, and velvety.
- It prepares the skin for makeup.
- It protects the skin from the pigments contained in makeup.

All this is not to say that a moisturizer "feeds" the skin externally. Skin is fed from within. A well-balanced diet provides nourishment to the skin's outermost cells.

There has been much controversy as to whether skin can be externally fed. This is really a matter of semantics. Perhaps, you can't feed your skin with nutrients, but your skin will definitely "drink!" Drinking is what we call absorption and the skin benefits from emollients and water. A complete moisturizer contains these ingredients in addition to those of its primary purpose, which is to form the external protective film. An under-makeup moisturizer concentrates on lubrication and leaves a little less film because makeup will join with it to form the protective film.

The skin's outermost cells are dead! The word dead implies to many of us "not having the capacity to do anything at all." Not true! The surface layers of the skin may be dead cells but they do hold water, steadily supplied from the sweat glands. It is the amount of water that these dead cells retain that is all-important to the skin's texture, color, and youthfulness. The surface layers of the skin also hold oil and it is this mixture of water and oil that forms the *acid mantle* for your skin's protection. A moisturizer doesn't physically moisturize the living inner layers within the skin's epidermis. A moisturizer is specifically designed to promote your own moisture by sealing in the available water, increasing and supplementing it to the outer layers.

A distinction must be made between the skin cells' ability to hold water and the pores that are the surface ends of the oil gland ducts. Pores are not cells and cells are not pores. Many, many women think their pores drink in moisturizing elements. They form a mental image of a moisturizer clogging up their pores. The

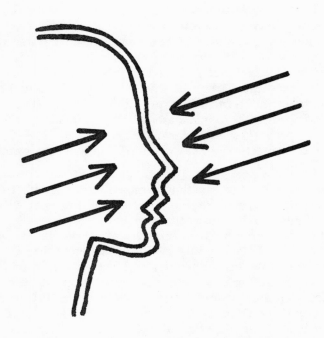

pores function is to excrete oil. It is the cells of the skin that form tissue—those fine 10 to 20 layers at the surface. These do the actual drinking or absorption. It is the outermost layers that need to be softened, lubricated, and protected. The only time you clog the pores, interspersed between the cells, is when you do not employ the proper cleansing methods, or if you put makeup on over dirty skin. Then the pores have the ability to grab and hold external dirt particles.

Moisturizing protection is the one and only effective method of protecting your skin from the outside elements, and of preventing water loss from within. It is this protection and prevention that slows down the aging process.

"Great!" you say, but all moisture escapes or evaporates. True! If you did nothing more, you would need to reapply your moisturizer every so often during the course of the day. But first you must wipe away the dirt the outside protective film has collected. This is where your skin freshener re-enters the picture, for few of us have the time or inclination during the day to start all over with the cleansing procedure. The freshener provides a fast and easy removal of the protective film along with the dirt and grime it has retained. If you were to neglect the skin freshener, the small dirt particles would be attracted into the pores. Remember, pores have the ability to grab and hold dirt as well as color.

BUT

There is a beautiful way to beat the system, without bothering to cleanse or reapply the moisturizer. In fact, you not only beat it, you improve upon it! You seal in the moisture of your moisturizer with a liquid or cream tinted foundation. Foundations contain varying amounts of moisturizers. By adding a tinted foundation to your moisturizer you achieve more benefits for your skin. You:

- eliminate the loss due to evaporation of your own moisture, while tripling the moisture protection;
- refine the appearance of your skin's texture;
- prepare the way for the color products of your makeup, permitting all of them to glide on more smoothly;
- even out the color of your skin; and
- freshen your appearance for a longer period of time.

Foundations will be further discussed in the makeup section of this book. But let's not get ahead of ourselves. We have quite a few more subjects to discuss, for while makeup can camouflage and improve, the quality of the skin beneath is most important. Even if you do not use makeup, a moisturizer itself will make the skin appear to be less lined and drawn, puffing up a certain amount of crepiness. A smooth flat surface reflects light more evenly than the irregular surface of even a slightly lined skin. The more moisture the skin retains, the more the skin puffs out to make fine lines far less noticeable. When you're over 30, this is a vital consideration.

NIGHT CREAMS AND LOTIONS: LET'S REALLY CLEAR UP THE CONFUSION!

Night creams and lotions are specially developed to be richer in emollients than most moisturizers. They protect the skin by relieving dryness and roughness. They help to promote smoothness and softness and they help considerably to retain the inner moisture in your skin. Their intended purpose is to remain in contact with the skin for an extended period of time—overnight!

It is believed that skin cells do most of their regenerating while you sleep. This renewal process is simultaneously building up a new supply of natural moisture within your skin. You want to retain that moisture, not lose it to the atmosphere, and it is the purpose of a night cream to *hold* it in.

Night creams and lotions are not miracle creams. There are no exotic, youth restoring or wrinkle remover ingredients contained in any cream or lotion, but they do have some beneficial ingredients that are absorbed by the skin. While the skin has a *barrier layer* just beneath the 10 to 20 layers of dead skin cells, the skin itself is not entirely a barrier. It has a selective ability to absorb a few specific cosmetic ingredients as well as medical ingredients.

While you may be somewhat disenchanted with the knowledge that there are no miracle creams, nonetheless, using night cream is a very important addition to your total skin care program.

The most important reason for using a night cream or lotion is to maintain and build your own inner moisture content by placing a shield (you might call it a mantle or a screen) between your face and the atmosphere in which you sleep, so that your inner moisture will not evaporate into the air. This is necessary, for no matter how ideal your bedroom atmosphere might be (a humidifier during winter, the steam heat months, would help to make it even more ideal), constant evaporation is taking place. For this reason, night creams should *not* be tissued off, even though the beneficial ingredients can be absorbed into your skin within twenty minutes.

This does not mean you need a thick glob of cream on your face, but you do need a heavier film to protect your face during the night, as it wears down while you naturally toss and turn on your pillow.

Speaking of pillows, did you know that the cumulative effect of burrowing your face in a pillow each night is a destructive force on its own? This can actually increase the furrows and folds of wrinkles, or create them! The constant friction and pressure, even though it is intermittent, due to tossing and turning, is simply too much pressure for your face. This action takes its effect little by little, contributing to the natural aging process.

The only way to get around this is to use a very small, soft pillow. Actually a baby pillow is ideal because it will support your head, but leave your face relatively free. Sleeping on your back all the time is another answer, but very few of us have that kind of body control while we sleep. Besides, that subject is in controversy: doctors now believe it is not good for the body to rest continually on the back during sleep. Another established fact is that if the head is lower than the feet it can cause puffiness under the eyes. Adequate elevation is a planned necessity. If a baby pillow does not give you enough height to support your head comfortably, put the baby pillow on top of your regular pillow, and instead of fluffing the pillow up, flatten it down. The two together will approximate the thickness of one fluffed pillow.

Almost paradoxically, relief of occasional swollen or puffy eyes is accomplished by lying down with your head lower than your shoulders and hips, while placing a few slices of raw potato or cotton saturated in milk over the swelling. Twenty minutes to half an hour usually does the trick.

The Extra-Dry Areas

For most skin types, a night cream is usually rich enough in emollients to use in the eye area as well as on the throat and neck. But, as you learned earlier, the skin in the eye area is exceedingly thin. An eye cream is a slightly modified emollient cream with perfume usually omitted. There is less subcutaneous fat in the skin around the eyes which also lacks natural oil glands. Therefore this is usually the first area to develop fine lines and wrinkles. Eye creams will not prevent wrinkles, but they help make these lines less noticeable because they are specifically formulated to penetrate this delicate eye area. For daytime, in addition to your moisturizer a wrinkle stick or eye gel or cream may be used under makeup to serve as a base for your eye makeup so it continually lubricates and plumps up the skin.

You will recall that everyone has far fewer *sebaceous* (oil) glands in the throat and neck area, therefore specific throat and neck creams are formulated to be extra rich to soften and smooth. They are usually heavier creams to permit a buildup of your own inner moisture by preventing its escape. These specialized creams are only necessary if your skin in these particular areas is extra-dry, lined or crepey.

And so, to Bed . . .

Let's talk about these necessary creams in relation to the men in our lives. There is absolutely no reason to present a greasy face to your man when you first go to bed. This is not the time to apply a

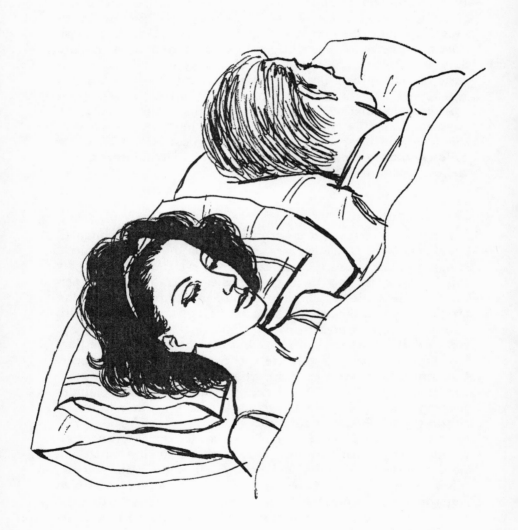

night cream so it is intact for the night. After the cleansing process, if you apply a light moisturizer to give your skin immediate protection, you will not appear or feel greasy. The richer, thicker night creams should be kept in your night table beside your bed and their application should be the very last thing you do before you go to sleep. You can even apply them in the dark . . . you know where your face is! Even if you forget the night cream occasionally, your previously applied moisturizer is giving your skin protection, though not as adequate as the night cream.

If you don't like going to bed with a completely nude face because you don't want your man to see it, here are some suggestions:

• Brush eyebrows to give them their most pleasing shape— give them the merest touch of eyebrow pencil if they need definition.

• Apply a slight touch of blue or grey liner or eyeshadow on your eyelids and use an eyelash conditioner, such as one of the automatic roll-on types, which besides conditioning gives the lashes more sheen, or use a bit of petroleum jelly to make the lashes glisten.

• Apply lip gloss or a chap preventive with a hint of color.

But remember, other than this your face is scrupulously clean and you have applied your moisturizer.

DISCIPLINING YOURSELF!

No regimen will work if you are not consistent. You must organize and discipline yourself to a daily schedule of morning and night cleansing. You can and will actually see the difference and the advantages in three to four weeks, and you can maintain this for the rest of your life.

All of the product types I have outlined and their progressive steps of use must be employed, for any one product without the other will not produce the glowing results. You must actually make a firm commitment to yourself, for skin can easily return to a dull state. Please remember, success is achieved by faithful, daily adherence to the cleansing routine which, I remind you, only takes three minutes.

In addition, try to set aside a special time at least once a week that you can call your very own. In that special time take care of all your beauty needs, whatever they may be.

Daily Cleansing Procedures

A FEW WORDS ABOUT PRODUCTS

The following daily procedures are classified by skin type as a guide to help you in your selection of products. This is by no means an all-inclusive list of brand names. There are other products made by different manufacturers that fall into the same categories. By writing to the manufacturer of your choice, if you are in doubt, you may determine their products for your skin type.

The majority of women over the age of 30 select one of the name brands represented here (but not necessarily the whole treatment line of any one company), as part of their cosmetic purchases. Of course, this does not always hold true and I apologize for any major omissions—they were not intentional. But general market acceptance and space within this book has made selection a necessity. You will find both lower and higher price ranges than those represented here. It is impossible to list them all.

There is admittedly a certain amount of overlapping of products among skin types. Some manufacturers consider certain of their products good for several different skin types. This has been taken into account in some cases but not necessarily in all, as the list then becomes boundless. In many instances I have placed that product in what I believe is the preferred skin type category which best serves the purpose of the consumer.

When selecting products for your individual skin type, make

71

sure you write the name in its entirety, exactly as you see it here. The difference of one word can indicate a totally different product within that company's line.

OILY SKIN

After precleansing to remove makeup, you should use a soap correlated to your specific oily condition. Use plenty of clear, warm to hot water, and then a high alcohol astringent type skin freshener. Apply a lightweight moisturizer if you have any dry patches. More than likely, you will need a moisturizer on your throat and neck and even perhaps over the entire face (see page 39) .

Morning and Night Routine

Use washcloth, buffing (**Buf-Puf**) or cleansing sponge, or complexion brush. Use gentle circular motions only. If time permits, a midday cleansing is advisable, or use special blotters to soak up excess oil especially designed for this purpose.

(All products in alphabetical order)

SOAPS TO USE:
Elizabeth Arden, Extra Benefit Soap for Oily Skin
Clearasil, Soap Developed for Oily Skin
Clinique, Facial Extra Strength for Oily Skin
Dial
Fostex Cake   (for acne-prone skin)
Glemby, Soft-Scrub Highly Efficient Soap
Hyperphase
Ivory
Jergens, Clear Complexion Bar
Lowilla Cake   (for sensitive, oily skin)
Neutrogena, Acne-Cleansing Soap   (for sensitive oily skin)
Phisoderm   (for sensitive, oily skin)
Pernox   (for active acne)
Revlon, Formula 2 Cleanser A

ASTRINGENTS TO USE:
Almay, Pore Lotion

Elizabeth Arden, Clarifying Astringent
Bonne Bell, Ten-O-Six Lotion
Clinique, Clarifying Lotion #3
DuBarry, Moisture Petals Oil-Vanishing Astringent
Etherea, Oil-Control Toning Lotion
Geminesse, Exhilarating Lotion
Glemby, Highly Efficient Astringent
Estée Lauder, Active Skin Lotion
Germaine Monteil, Clarifying Astringent
Helena Rubinstein, Skin Life Bracing Astringent
Ultima, Skim Milk Fresh Purifying Tonic

MOISTURIZERS TO USE:
DuBarry, Moisture Petals Oil-Vanishing Moisturizer
Geminesse, Under Makeup Moisturizing Tint (Natural)
Estée Lauder, Non-Oily Under Makeup Cream
Germaine Monteil, Clarity Oil Free Moisture for Day & Night
Pond's, Vanishing Cream
Revlon, Formula 2 Moisturizer A
Shiseido, Oil Blotting Moisture Lotion
Ultima, Skim Milk Fresh Daily Moisture
Vaseline, Intensive Care

NORMAL COMBINATION SKIN

Type I: Normal to Oily

To achieve maximum positive results, this type of skin has to be treated as though you owned two different faces.

After precleansing to remove makeup, you should use a mild soap and plenty of clear, lukewarm water (15 to 20 splashes are enough). Then use a medium alcohol content skin freshener on the drier portions of your face, and a more astringent type (higher alcohol content) freshener on your T-zone. (If the drier areas of your face are very dry, see page 79 and use one of the skin fresheners under the heading of "Dry Skin.") Follow with a lightweight moisturizer. Reverse the skin freshener procedure if your T-zone is dry and the sides of your face are oily.

Morning and Night Routine

Use washcloth or fingertips on the drier areas of your face. Within the T-zone area, use buffing (**Buf-Puf**) or cleansing sponge or a complexion brush. Use gentle circular motions.

(*All products in alphabetical order*)

SOAPS TO USE:
Camay
Dove
Hyperphase
Ivory
Lux
Neutrogena Regular or Acne-Cleansing
Phisoderm
Vel Beauty Bar

STRONGER SKIN FRESHENERS TO USE WITHIN THE T-ZONE AREA:
Almay, Pore Lotion
Elizabeth Arden, Clarifying Astringent
Borghese, Balancing & Toning Lotion (Normal to Oily)
Clinique, Clarifying Lotion #3
Etherea, Oil Control Toning Lotion
Geminesse, Toning Lotion
Dorothy Gray, Texture Lotion
Lancôme, Fraicheur Tonique
Estée Lauder, Active Skin Lotion
Germaine Monteil, Super Tone Skin Conditioner
Helena Rubinstein, Skin Life Bracing Astringent
Ultima, Skim Milk Purifying Tonic

MILDER SKIN FRESHENERS TO USE OUTSIDE OF T-ZONE AREA:
Almay, Deep Mist Toning & Refining Lotion
Elizabeth Arden, Skin Lotion
Borghese, Balancing & Toning Lotion (Normal to Dry)
Clinique, Clarifying Lotion #2
Coty, Equasion Balancing Toner
Etherea, Balanced Toning Lotion
Fabergé, Babe Fabulous Freshener

Geminesse, Moisturizing Skin Freshener
Dorothy Gray, Orange Flower Skin Freshener
Estée Lauder, Skin Lotion
Germaine Monteil, Skin Freshener
Helena Rubinstein, Skin Life Toning Refreshant
Ultima II, Skim Milk Fresh Purifying Toner

MOISTURIZERS TO USE:
Geminesse, Under Makeup Moisturizer
Lancôme, Bienfait Du Matin Conditioning Daytime Creme
Estée Lauder, Non-Oily Under Makeup Cream
Germaine Monteil, Regime Emulsified Moisture
Helena Rubinstein, Fresh Cover Cool Moisture
Ultima II, Skim Milk Fresh Daily Moisture

Type II: Normal

After precleansing to remove makeup, you should use a mild soap, plenty of lukewarm, clear water rinses, and a medium alcohol content skin freshener. Then use a lightweight moisturizer.

Morning and Night Routine

Use washcloth and/or fingertips. A Buf-Puf or complexion brush may be used occasionally. Use gentle circular motions only. *(All products in alphabetical order)*

SOAPS TO USE:
Camay
Cashmere Bouquet
Dove
Ivory
Jergens
Lux
Neutrogena, Regular
Palmolive, Regular (not gold)
Tone

SKIN FRESHENERS TO USE:
Almay, Deep Mist Toning & Refining Lotion
Elizabeth Arden, Skin Lotion
Borghese, Clean Skin Simply Toner
Charles of the Ritz, Double Phase Rousing Toner
Clinique, Clarifying Lotion #2
Coty, Equasion Balancing Toner
Etherea, Balanced Toning Lotion
Fabergé, Babe Fabulous Freshener
Halston, Toner
Estée Lauder, Skin Lotion
Germaine Monteil, Skin Freshener
Helena Rubinstein, Skin Life Toning Refreshant
Ultima II, Skim Milk Fresh Purifying Toner

MOISTURIZERS TO USE:
Elizabeth Arden, Velva Moisture Film
Borghese, Clean Skin Simply Moisturizer AM/PM
Coty, Equasion Fresh Peach Moisture Cream
Etherea, Maximum Moisturizer
Fabergé, Babe Dewy Moisturizer
Halston, Moisturizer
Jergens, Facial Moisture Cream
Lancôme, Frescabel Pre-Makeup Emulsion
Estée Lauder, Lightweight Re-Nutriv Creme
Germaine Monteil, Bio-Miracle Lotion
Pond's, Light Moisturizer Under Make-up Conditioner
Revlon, Moon Drops Undermakeup Moisture Film
Helena Rubinstein, Skin Life Lightweight Emulsion
Ultima II, Under Makeup Moisture Lotion

Type III: Normal to Dry

As in the case of the Normal to Oily, this type skin also has to be treated as though you owned two different faces to achieve maximum results.

After precleansing to remove makeup, you should use a mild soap, plenty of clear, lukewarm water rinses (20 splashes are enough), and follow with a mild alcohol content skin freshener on the drier portions of your face and a slightly higher alcohol content freshener on your T-zone. (If the oily areas of your face are very oily, see page 74 and use one of the skin fresheners under the heading of "stronger skin fresheners for Normal to Oily skin.") Follow with a medium-weight moisturizer.

Morning and Night Routine

Use washcloth or fingertips on drier areas. A complexion brush or buffing (**Buf-Puf**) or cleansing sponge may be used occasionally. Use gentle circular motions only.
(All products in alphabetical order)

SOAPS TO USE:
Aveeno Bar
Basis
Camay
Cashmere Bouquet
Dove
Jergens
Lowilla Cake
Lux
Neutrogena, Regular
Oilatum
Palmolive, Regular (not gold)
Tone

SKIN FRESHENERS TO USE:
Almay, Deep Mist Mild Freshener
Elizabeth Arden, Velva Smooth Lotion
Borghese, Balancing & Toning Lotion (Normal to Dry)
Clinique, Clarifying Lotion #1
Coty, Equasion Balancing Freshener
Geminesse, Moisturizing Skin Freshener
Dorothy Gray, Orange Flower Skin Freshener
Germaine Monteil, Acti-Vita Cream Toner
Ultima II, Gentle Skin Balancing Lotion

SLIGHTLY STRONGER SKIN FRESHENERS TO USE WITHIN THE T-ZONE AREA:
Almay, Deep Mist Toning & Refining Lotion
Elizabeth Arden, Skin Lotion

Borghese, Balancing & Toning Lotion (Normal to Oily)
Clinique, Clarifying Lotion #2
Coty, Equasion Balancing Toner
Etherea, Balanced Toning Lotion
Fabergé, Great Skin with NMC-12 Freshener
Geminesse, Toning Lotion
Dorothy Gray, Texture Lotion
Germaine Monteil, Super Moist Toning Lotion
Ultima II, Lotion Refreshant

MOISTURIZERS TO USE:
Almay, Deep Mist Ultralight, Moisture Lotion for Combination to Slightly Dry Skin
Elizabeth Arden, Velva Moisture Film
Borghese, Beauty Treatment Moisturizer
Clinique, Dramatically Different Moisturizing Lotion
Coty, Vitamin Moisture Balancer
Fabergé, Great Skin with NMC-12 Day Care Moisturizer
Geminesse, Enriched Moisturizing Complex Lotion
Estée Lauder, Daily Moisture Supply Lotion
L'Oréal, Aqualia Moisture Equalizer
Noxzema, Raintree Moisture Maker (Normal to Dry)
Orlane, Crème Hydratante Fluide
Revlon, Moon Drops Under Makeup Moisture Balm
Helena Rubinstein, Moisture Response
Scandia, Artesian Basic Moisturizer
Toni, division of Gillette, Deep Magic Lotion
Ultima, Skim Milk Fresh Daily Moisture for Normal to Slightly Dry Skin

DRY SKIN

Night Routine

After precleansing to remove makeup, you should use a very mild or superfatted soap, or a rinsable cleanser. Use extra soft washcloth or fingertips. You may occasionally use a buffing (Buf-Puf) or cleansing sponge lightly. Use gentle circular motions only. Rinse with 20 splashes of lukewarm water. Follow with a very mild low alcohol content skin freshener (witch hazel may be substituted), and then follow with a rich emollient moisturizer.

Morning Routine

Omit soap or rinsable cleanser procedure. Cleanse your face with lukewarm water using your fingertips or extra soft washcloth. Use gentle circular motions only. Pat dry. Wipe your face gently with skin freshener and then moisturize.
(All products in alphabetical order)

SOAPS TO USE:
Aveeno Bar
Basis
Dove
Lowilla Cake
Neutrogena, Dry-Skin
Nivea
Oilatum
Tone

RINSABLE CLEANSERS TO USE:
Elizabeth Arden, Milky Cleanser
Max Factor, Facial Bath
Lancôme, Ablutia
Pond's, Creamy Facial Cleanser
Revlon, Eterna 27 Daily Care Cleansing Bar for Dry and
    Delicate Skin
Tussy, Happy Face
Ultima II, Milk Bath

SKIN FRESHENERS TO USE:
Almay, Deep Mist Mild Freshener
Elizabeth Arden, Velva Smooth Lotion
Borghese, Toning Lotion for Dry Skin
Clinique, Clarifying Lotion #1
Coty, Equasion Balancing Freshener
Calvin Klein, Skin Plan II Night Toner
Germaine Monteil, Acti-Vita Pure Cream Toner
Orlane, Tonique Freshener
Ultima II, Gentle Skin-Balancing Lotion

MOISTURIZERS TO USE:
Elizabeth Arden, Visible Difference Refining Moisture
    Creme Complex

Biersdorf, Nivea Skin Cream
Marian Bialac, Yatrolin L'Quide Moisturizing Lotion
Charles of the Ritz, Revenescence Liquid
Clinique, Dramatically Different Moisturizing Lotion or Concentrate
Jacqueline Cochran, Flowing Velvet Hydrophilic Lotion
Coty, One Perfect Ounce
Frances Denny, Multi-Layer Moisturizer
Doak, Formula 405 Light Textured Moisturizer
Calvin Klein, Skin Plan II, Moisturizing Lotion
Estée Lauder, Estoderm Flowing Emulsion
Germaine Monteil, Acti-Vita Enriched Moisturizer
Noxzema, Raintree Moisture Maker for Dry Skin
Olay, Oil of Olay
Revlon, Eterna 27 All-Day Moisture Lotion or Cream
Helena Rubinstein, Skin Dew Visible Action Moisturizing Emulsion
Scandia, Kvalia Day Cream Formula
Irma Shorell, Moisture/35
Syntex, Lotion for Dry Skin
Texas Pharmaceuticals, Lubriderm
Toni, division of Gillette, Deep Magic Moisturizer Cream

VERY DRY, SENSITIVE OR DELICATE SKIN

Method I

After precleansing to remove makeup, you should use a very mild soap or rinsable cleanser with just enough lukewarm, clear rinsing water to remove the film. A rinsable cleanser is more difficult to remove than soap because it does not lather, so extra care is advised.

Method II

Your alternative is to use a cleansing cream specifically formulated for sensitive skin, which is tissued off and the excess is gently wiped away with several pieces of cotton saturated in skin freshener.

With either method, follow with a very mild skin freshener to remove every last trace of residue. Then follow with an emollient moisturizer formulated for sensitive, delicate skin. It may also be advisable to apply the moisturizer twice, waiting five minutes between applications.

Use either of the above procedures for both morning and night applications. Use an extra soft washcloth and/or your fingertips in featherlike circular movements on your face. Gently pat dry.

If you have any oily patches, see page 37.

(All products in alphabetical order)

SOAPS TO USE:
Alpha Keri
Aveeno Bar
Formula 405
Lowilla Cake
Neutrogena, Unscented or Dry-Skin
Oilatum

RINSABLE CLEANSERS TO USE:
Elizabeth Arden, Milky Cleanser
Max Factor, Facial Bath
Lancôme, Ablutia
Pond's, Creamy Facial Cleanser
Revlon, Eterna 27 Daily Care Cleansing Bar for Dry and Delicate Skin
Tussy, Happy Face
Ultima II, Milk Bath

SKIN FRESHENERS TO USE:
Elizabeth Arden, Fragile Skin Toner
Pier Augé, Leapsal Tonic Peau Sèche Dry and Sensitive Skin
Borghese, Balancing & Toning Lotion for Dry Delicate Skin
Charles of the Ritz, Gentle Toning Lotion
Essentia, Skin Refining Tonic
Orlane, Ligne Integrale Special Lotion Sans Alcool

MOISTURIZERS TO USE:
Christian Dior, Hydra Dior Base Protectrice
Essentia, Protective Moisture Lotion for Delicate Skin
Geminesse, Enriched Moisturizing Complex Cream
Estée Lauder, Swiss Performing Extract
Orlane, Ligne Integrale Creme de Jour Moisturizer
Texas Pharmaceuticals, Lubriderm

ULTRA-DRY (DEHYDRATED) SKIN

Morning and Night Routine

You should cleanse your face with a cleansing cream or lotion especially formulated for ultra-dry or dehydrated skin. Tissue it off gently and then repeat the application. You might try alternating this procedure with soap and water or rinsable cleanser once or twice a week progressing to three times a week.

Use a specially formulated skin freshener for your skin type (preferably one containing no alcohol). Repeat with several applications of cotton saturated freshener until the last cotton ball looks completely clean.

Follow immediately with a very rich moisturizer for daytime and/or a night cream, again formulated for your skin type. It may also be advisable to apply these emollient creams twice, waiting five minutes between applications.

Use fingertips only in featherlike circular movements on your face when applying any product. If you are extremely dehydrated consultant a physician or dermatologist.

(All products in alphabetical order)

SOAPS TO USE:
Alpha Keri
Aveeno Bar
Formula 405
Lowilla Cake
Neutrogena, Dry-Skin or Baby Soap
Oilatum

RINSABLE CLEANSERS TO USE:
Elizabeth Arden, Milky Cleanser

Max Factor, Facial Bath
Lancôme, Ablutia
Pond's, Creamy Facial Cleanser
Revlon, Eterna 27 Daily Care Cleansing Bar for Dry
      and Delicate Skin
Tussy, Happy Face
Ultima II, Milk Bath

CLEANSING CREAMS TO USE:
Christian Dior, Lait Démaquillant Hydratant Moisturizing
      Cleanser
Max Factor, Pure Moisture Lotion Cleanser
Geminesse, Enriched Moisturizing Cleansing Concentrate
Lancôme, Douceur Démaquillante Nutrix Cleansing Creme

SKIN FRESHENERS TO USE:
Christian Dior, Lotion de Fraicheur (no alcohol)
Max Factor, Ultralucent Pure Moisture Refining Toner
Geminesse, Enriched Moisturizing Skin Freshener
Lancôme, Tonique Douceur (no alcohol)
Helena Rubinstein, Skin Life Deep Moisture Alcohol-Free
      Freshener
Diane Von Furstenberg, Freshener (no alcohol)

MOISTURIZERS TO USE:
Almay, Deep-Mist, Ultrarich Moisture Cream For Extra-
   Dry Skin
Alo-Cosmetics, After Tan Moisturizing Lotion
Beiersdorf, Nivea Skin Oil
Borghese, Crema Concentrata Moisturizing Creme
Charles of the Ritz, Cream Revenescence
Christian Dior, Hydra Dior Creme Extra Riche
Clinique, Dramatically Different Moisturizing Concentrate
Doak, Formula 405 Deep-Action Moisturizer Cream
Max Factor, Ultralucent Moisture Cream Concentrate
Geminesse, Living Proof Hydracel Moisturizer Cream
Lancôme, Hydrix and/or Lancomia
Noxzema, Raintree Concentrated Moisture Maker for Extra
      Dry Skin
Orlane, Creme Hydratant Fluide
Helena Rubinstein, Existence Poly-Active Cream

THREE-MINUTE
NIGHTLY ACTION CAPSULE
(STEP-BY-STEP REVIEW)

1. Remove makeup and dirt with precleansing cream or lotion. Tissue off in upward, outward motions (this applies to all following steps) .

2. Wash face and neck with soap and lukewarm water (or rinsable cleanser) using washcloth, fingertips, etc., for about 30 seconds. Rinse in clear lukewarm water, splashing no more than one minute.

3. Gently pat face dry using fresh towel. Do not rub.

4. Wash eyes with cotton that is well saturated in eyewash. Wash from inside corner to outside using fresh cotton for each eye.

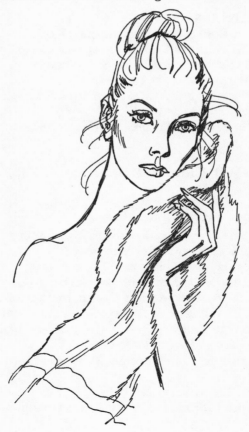

5. Wipe entire face and neck (excluding eyes) with cotton saturated with skin freshener. (If combination skin requiring two fresheners, use stronger one first.) Wipe until cotton looks clean. Use another cotton saturated ball if necessary, but continue until cotton looks clean. Allow to dry for a few moments. Alcohol content evaporates quickly and when the tingle subsides . . .

6. Apply moisturizer. Put five generous dots on each of following: forehead, cheeks, nose, and chin. Place another two dots on neck. Spread evenly and gently with upward, outward motions using fingertips. Do not rub. Use featherlike strokes in eye area.

7. Apply richer emollient cream when you are in bed and are ready to go to sleep.

Morning Action Capsule: Repeat steps 2 through 6.

SUPPLEMENTING YOUR SKIN'S CLEANSING PROGRAM

There are other extremely important cleansing techniques that are basic to a healthy, radiant, glowing skin. These techniques, which supplement the daily cleansing routine, are usually employed on a once-a-week basis (twice, if you can manage it). These procedures are not to be avoided or considered a sometime treat. They are truly essential and not a luxury. Exfoliants and/or masks are the final steps that contribute to the overall cleansing plan that definitely makes the difference between good skin and glorious skin. These procedures fit into the hour that is specifically your time, that we talked about earlier.

After 30 the outer layers of the skin tend to be drier, have increased pigmentation, are usually blotchy, and have cellular buildup (thickened, dead skin cells).

Naturally this buildup interferes with the texture, color, and contour of your skin. (Regardless of skin type, the universal outcry is, "But I have large pores! What can I do?" Exfoliants do answer this need also.) Before 30, the skin quite naturally sheds the dead skin cells, but now the cells stick together much more readily. The continuous surface cast-off simply slows down after 30. You have to help shed the buildup of these thickened, coarsened cells that appear as thick skin (with or without fine crepy lines and/or roughness).

Exfoliation

Exfoliation is the act of using an abrasive skin cleanser especially formulated for the job. Its purpose is to rid the skin of the accumulation of dead skin cells that adhere to the surface and which would not otherwise be removed by normal daily cleansing. The buildup makes the skin look dull, dry, and coarse.

Exfoliants come in many different forms. These relatively unknown products have instantaneous beneficial effects. There is no doubt they are the greatest skin beautifiers we have at our disposal. Dull looking skin is due to the non-use of this type product. Every woman needs an exfoliator and/or mask, because we do not get the daily benefits, as men do, from shaving. A man's skin benefits daily, because he is shaving off the dead skin cells of the outermost layers. Men are subject to a cellular buildup, but it is more vigorously removed with each and every shave. That's the reason that many men have younger looking skin than their wives.

Exfoliating your skin should be done once a week, twice if you think you can tolerate it. Actually, the best plan is to use an abrasive exfoliant once and switch to a mask for your second weekly deep cleansing. Instructions come with each product and should be read thoroughly and followed to the letter as there are several different types. Be sure to remove every last trace and follow with moisturizer.

Any exfoliating product with an abrasive action will get the job done. Here are some of them:

(in alphabetical order)

Elizabeth Arden, Skin Dynamics Complexion Renewal Lotion
Clinique, 7th Day Scrub or Exfoliating Lotion for Oily Skin
Max Factor, Swedish Formula Purified Cleansing Grains (Dry Skin)
Estée Lauder, Solid Milk Cleansing Grains
Germaine Monteil, Clarity Beauty Beads or Facial Sluffing Cream
Helena Rubinstein, Beauty Washing Grains
Irma Shorell, Dermabrase/35
Ultima, Clarifying Cleansing Wash

Masks

Masks are terrific cleansers in addition to the regular cleansing routine and the exfoliating process. They too slough off dead skin cells and sweep away some impurities from the skin's surface, but to a lesser degree than the more abrasive type exfoliating product, so they really should not take the place of it.*

But the mask offers something that the exfoliator cannot—that is, it forms a watertight shield on your face to permit a rich natural moisture build-up within your skin, during the time it is worn. It is the water in your skin that keeps it soft and smooth and prevents wrinkles! The mask also temporarily tightens the pores while firming the skin, which lasts a few hours. Masks activate circulation which helps to cleanse away toxic matter, the cause of spots and dull skin tone. Your skin feels revitalized and the pores appear to be refined. And masks have an extra plus: they encourage you to relax!

A mask may be used as often as once a day for all skin types, but most of us are lucky if we can find time once or twice a week. It is a good habit to get into. Remember, "Your time." Make it as often as you like.

There are many and various forms of masks. Gels are the most gentle and are rinsed off with water. The refreshing pick-me-up types are usually the peel-off variety. Moisturizing masks are in the thick facial category and deep cleansing masks contain additional abrasives. Have your beauty advisor or cosmetician help you select, as they should be purchased according to your skin type; one more reason to know exactly what your skin type is. (See pages 31 to 42.)

Here are some of them. For the most part, they are in the deep cleansing category, according to individual skin type.

(In alphabetical order)

Elizabeth Arden, Velva   Normal to dry
Cream Mask

---

* Exception is the mature woman with sensitive and delicate skin. (See page 37.) Also black women, see pages 39–41, and women in general who have extremely sensitive, delicate skin.

Borghese, Beauty Treatment Clay Masque	Oily skin
Charles of the Ritz, Revene-scence Revitalizing Masque	Normal to dry
Clinique, Beauty Emer-gency Masque	Normal to oily
Christian Dior, Hydra Dior Masque	Very dry or dehydrated skin
Essentia, Moisture Rescue Pack Firming Mask	Sensitive, delicate dry skin
Lancôme, Absolue Masque #10	Normal to oily
Estée Lauder, Almond Clay Pack	Oily skin
Germaine Monteil, Acti-Vita Peel-Off Masque Facial	Dry skin
Revlon, Moisturizing Honey Pack	Dry skin
Helena Rubinstein, Bio-Clear Medicated Mask	Oily problem skin
Shiseido, Facial Pack	Dry skin
Ultima, Creme Masque Con-centrate	Oily skin

Facial Saunas:
Who Should Use Them and Who Shouldn't?

To be effective, saunas really have to be hot! Physicians and der-matologists recognize that extreme water temperatures—too much hot or too much cold—can be a shock to the skin, especially in women over 30. Shock or trauma can disrupt fine capillaries that lie very close to the skin's surface, causing little red lines or web-like spots on the skin.

Using facial saunas, therefore, becomes a questionable matter. Certainly women with sensitive, delicate skin could not possibly tolerate the intense heat in the first place. Women with dry skin may find it difficult to stay under long enough to get substantial hydrating benefits, although the woman who has a tougher, sun-thickened, dehydrated skin may very well find it beneficial. Even the normal and combination skins are taking a risk by using facial saunas that doesn't seem proportionate to the temporary hydrating benefits. Now we come to the woman who has oily skin, the skin that is oily all over. It is true that this type of skin can take somewhat more punishment because it is thicker and coarser. Also, since the pores are usually larger, the intense heat of the sauna has the ability to reduce coarseness, loosen up clogs, and may wash them away. Facial saunas are advisable for hydrating the sun-thickened, dehydrated skin (if one uses a very emollient cream immediately afterward) and for the woman with overall oily skin. But, women with oily skin should use an astringent immediately afterward to remove the excess sebum and help further tighten up the forced enlargement of the pores.

To those women who have dry, normal, and combination skins, all I can say is, "Use your common sense in light of these facts," but never use a facial sauna for more than ten minutes in one session.

A SPECIAL NOTE TO THE MATURE WOMAN

Lined skin is more than likely dry to very dry skin. It will benefit greatly from exfoliation to remove dead skin cells that make its texture look flaky, drab, or dull, and it is much more easily moisturized.

Scrubbing grains in a rinsable cleansing cream will leave no drying effect. Another type of exfoliator is a gel which is peeled off in one piece. If these types prove to be too harsh, there are gel masks that form a clear film that is rinsed off with water. Herbal masks are also gentle. These may be best for older, more deeply lined skin. Clay masks are too oil absorbing and not as kind.

In addition to exfoliants, I would like to bring to your attention certain products that appear to plump up lined skin. They form a smooth invisible surface on your face and their clear films are usually worn under tinted foundation to reflect light more evenly in order to give it the appearance of fewer lines. Several such products are:

(in alphabetical order)

Elizabeth Arden, Bye-Lines Undermakeup Wrinkle Lotion
Lancôme, Adieu Rides Wrinkle Creme
Estée Lauder, European Performing Creme
Germaine Monteil, Acti-Vita Line Smoothing Formula
Ultima, Translucent Wrinkle Lotion

If you are contemplating cosmetic surgery, you should know that all cleansing and makeup procedures in this book are medically approved by plastic surgeons. Of course, you need permission from your doctor to use them, which usually can be done two weeks after surgery.

Special Facial Beauty Procedures

LET'S HAVE A CLEAR UNDERSTANDING OF BLACKHEADS, WHITEHEADS AND PIMPLES

A blackhead (*comedo*) is a plug of hardened oil that lies at the top of the follicle, plugging up the pore. It started out as a waxy matter having a light color. Since the skin did not close over it, the opening at the surface has permitted the plug to oxidize (the effect of oxygen in the air), producing a brownish-black color. This is not dirt or soil from the atmosphere. Upon removal and examination, it has a cone shape with the narrow end of the cone still retaining a light color and waxy appearance. These plugs come from *within*. The follicle has been plugged up with dried oil matter and is backing up the normal flow of oil to the skin's surface.

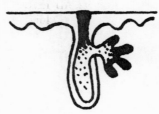

A whitehead (*milia*) is an accumulation of dead skin cells and sebum formed into a hardened, waxy plug enclosed by a fine layer of skin. Since it is not exposed to the air, it has not had the opportunity to oxidize. Whiteheads may or may not become pimples, but they may become larger and are sometimes subject to infection. Usually they do not disappear with time or with normal cleansing procedures.

It is more difficult to remove a whitehead than a blackhead because it is enclosed. The fine layer of skin must be punctured with a sterile needle in order to expose it. *Do not use pins.* Needles are manufactured differently and you need the extra sharpness and better metal to expose the whitehead for removal.

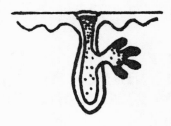

A pimple (*pustule*) is an irritated blackhead or whitehead that has been allowed to advance to the next stage, to flourish in bacteria and go unattended. It is larger in size and appears to be bulging with impurities and foreign matter. Here there is the com-

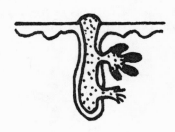

plete closure of the sebaceous (oil) gland preventing the sebum's flow to the surface. This is usually accompanied by some redness in the immediate surrounding area.

A cyst differs from a pimple in that it is larger in size, deeper, and the immediate surrounding area is highly inflamed. This is a hard painful lump and lasts much longer than even a severe pimple. A cyst is definitely a case for your physician or dermatologist, for it requires medical treatment. If you have a prolonged eruption at the time of this reading and it seems to fit the above description, do not assume it is a pimple. You must make the assumption that it is more serious and put yourself in the care of a doctor.

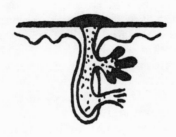

Acne

All of the preceding conditions are simple and occasional problems and are not to be confused with what is known as adult acne. The term acne covers the vast realm of all outbreaks of the skin, even merely one blackhead or whitehead.

Please remember that this book was written for women over the age of 30. Above all, resist the temptation to apply the methods and techniques that follow to your teenage children. Their external skin outbreaks and blemishes are due to various stages of acne, which are basically due to a hormone imbalance peculiar to adolescents and some adults. This is quite different from what we are discussing here. If you have an excessive quantity of pimples and you are over 30, do not deal with them as I have outlined. You should check with a dermatologist because it is an abnormal condition at this stage of life.

Acne scars can be removed even after 30. Consult a dermatologist. You may have a wonderful surprise in store for you. There are new techniques that are not as expensive or time consuming as they once were, and which can remove even deep craters. But, be realistic! Some women expect to have the skin of a newborn baby. Even if you can only achieve a 50 percent improvement, that's a lot!

Dealing with Blackheads, Whiteheads, and Pimples

Now that you have a working knowledge and a mental picture of what these conditions are, we can deal with them. Everyone gets an occasional blackhead, whitehead, or pimple, but you should also understand that a skin eruption at or about the time of your menstrual period or associated with it in any way should be left alone. The blood stream will clear it. If, for some reason, it does not clear up in a reasonable period of time, you should see your gynecologist or dermatologist to determine if anything is medically wrong. If any pimple, regardless of its cause, does not appear to be bulging with matter, let nature take its course.

For purposes of clarity, we will call a blackhead or whitehead a *plug* because it plugs up from within due to an overactive oil gland. Dirt and grime we'll label a *clog* because it is attracted into the pores from without and results in what appears to be a blackhead but is due to improper and inadequate cleansing.

In the future, you are highly unlikely to get clogs when you follow the proper cleansing procedures. A plug from within can happen, but its incidence is also reduced with thorough cleansing and the use of masks or exfoliators as well as saunas. In any case, all of these methods will help loosen them. It may be difficult for you to determine whether they are from within or without. It does not matter, they are both treated alike after all cleansing procedures have been utilized. If they are clogs, a thorough cleansing might wash them away. This is why it is advantageous to assume they are clogs until proven otherwise with one of the above mentioned cleansing procedures.

Here's your plan of action: Your magnifying mirror (preferably lighted) is essential here. You will need a blackhead remover, also known as a comedo extractor. It is a medically approved, inexpensive item and it may be purchased at a surgical supply house or your local drugstore. If the druggist doesn't carry it in stock, he will order it for you. Try to get the best one possible and look for or ask for one that has good curves extending from its center handle. One that is too flat can be troublesome because it forces you to exert undue pressure.

Never, never use your fingernails or fingertips. Besides being unsterile, they are just too big and cumbersome for this delicate operation and do not offer you the necessary control. Please, either do it properly or let your dermatologist do it for you. The only reason I include this procedure in this book is because I find very few of us running to the dermatologist every time we get a black-head!

At this point, we will assume you have gone through the entire cleansing procedure:

1. Precleansed with your cleansing cream or lotion.

2. Washed your face with soap and water, rinsed adequately in clear, clean water.

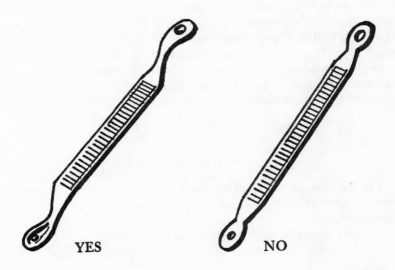

YES   NO

A comedo extractor is a small instrument with rounded ends.
Each end has a hole—one smaller and one slightly larger

3. Exfoliated the skin with a product made specifically for that purpose, or used a mask or a sauna.

4. Wiped away all last traces with your skin freshener or astringent. (Do not apply moisturizer in this case.)

Now you find you may have some blackheads and perhaps also a few whiteheads. [Note: The following treatment is for all skin types except the sensitive and dehydrated.] To those with all other skin types please remember not to treat more than three blemishes at one time and they should not be within ¼ inch (preferably ½ inch) in distance from each other. If there are more, save them for another day. You've lived with them this long, they will wait a bit longer for the sake of preventing irritation or redness. I realize there is a temptation to try to extract all of the blemishes with a new found knowledge and method, but moderation is the keynote, besides being the safest way to go. Incidentally, the method is *not new*. It's just one of those "closet" subjects that no one cares to discuss.

Please remember, not to overtreat. Overtreating is applying undue pressure more than twice on the same pore on the same day. To persist in extraction is folly (especially with pimples) and will only cause irritation and perhaps force the contents into the surrounding tissue. If any blackhead, whitehead, or pimple does not remove easily, do not force. Take heart in knowing you have succeeded in causing the blemish to rise and somewhat loosen. Undoubtedly, you will be successful when you try in another day or two, but always observe the same sterile conditions.

Sterilizing the Blackhead Extractor

The blackhead extractor must be sterilized first. There are three ways to sterilize, any of which are acceptable by medical standards. Choose one.

• Submerge in boiling water for 15 minutes.

• Immerse in 70 percent alcohol (rubbing alcohol) for 30 minutes.

• Flame both ends for a few seconds with a match or cigarette lighter. Remove black carbon deposits with alcohol-saturated cotton. Wipe thoroughly.

IMPORTANT NOTE: Touch and hold only the center handle for all three methods.

Extracting Blackheads, Whiteheads, and Pimples

Apply a hot compress for five minutes to the immediate area of the blackhead to help loosen the internal matter. One or two cotton balls wrung out in very hot tap water will keep the compress localized. The cotton is small and gives you complete control. There is no need to shock other areas of the face.

With a fresh cotton ball or pad saturated in 70 percent alcohol (rubbing alcohol) dab the pore and its immediate surrounding area.

You are now ready to use the blackhead remover. Place the end with the SMALLER hole over the blackhead and center the hole directly on it. When you have made certain that you are exactly on target, exert a quick, firm pressure ever so slightly to the side. This should release the matter into the hole of the blackhead remover. Redab the area with alcohol saturated cotton. If the matter did not release, it may mean that you were not centered properly and you may try once more.

After you have extracted the impurity, dab the treated area with alcohol. Now clean the head of the blackhead remover with a clean tissue corner twisted to a fine point and dip it in alcohol. Put it right through the hole until it will go no further and tear the rest of the tissue off. The twisted end of the tissue will retain the extracted matter. This serves two purposes: (1) You are re-sterilizing the inside hole of the blackhead remover; (2) you can examine the extracted matter to give you a good idea as to the state of your skin and the cleansing methods you have employed in the past. If the matter was cone-shaped, it was a plug of dried oil. If not, it was a clog due to improper cleansing.

A whitehead is treated in exactly the same manner except you must add a step if you see that it is covered with a fine layer of skin. Some are not, they are the very beginning of a blackhead which as yet has not oxidized to give it the dark color.

• Sterilize the tip of a fine needle (no pins please) under the flame of a match for a few seconds. Wipe the needle tip

with alcohol saturated cotton to remove the black carbon.
• Dab the whitehead with alcohol saturated cotton.
• Center the tip of needle on the enclosed whitehead and puncture it.
• Proceed with instructions for blackhead removal, using the *smaller* of the two holes.

A pimple is treated in exactly the same manner as a whitehead, except you use the *larger* of the two holes. After the initial pus matter is removed, turn the extractor over and use the smaller hole once more to remove the secondary matter that is lying in the follicle. Most likely, you have removed the entire impurity, but if not, wait another day or two and repeat the procedure if the skin does not appear to be flat where the matter was removed. The deeply seated secondary matter will rise on its own and then you will most likely be successful.

Make sure to wipe with alcohol on each successive removal of pus matter, and then give it a final dab with alcohol saturated cotton. Do not use foundation makeup and avoid moisturizer in that particular area for at least one day.

Alternative Method for Dealing with Pimples

There is another way of treating a pimple other than physically extracting it. There are medicated ointments which are available at your local drugstore that will make the pimple dry and peel.
(*In alphabetical order*)

Acne-Aid	(Stiefel)
Clearasil	(Vicks)
Oxy 5	(Norcliff-Thayer)
Phisoac	(Winthrop)
Transact	(Westwood)
Vanoxide	(Dermik)

If you are squeamish about applying these measures to yourself and you see blemishes or eruptions of the type we have previously discussed, then by all means see a dermatologist. You don't want them to develop into more serious pimples.

This is not a common situation, but you should know that there is an area known as the "triangle of death." This refers to a triangle between the eyebrows and the lower points just above the corners of the mouth, encompassing the area on either side of the nose. It has long been recognized as an area of the face where one should not squeeze on the theory that an infection from this area (the veins of which drain into the cavernous sinus just below the brain) can be fatal. While it is rare, it has happened.

ACTION CAPSULE

(Step-by-Step Review)

MATERIALS NEEDED:
Magnifying mirror (if not lighted, place in a strong light)
Blackhead remover
Alcohol (70% ethyl rubbing alcohol)
Cotton balls or pads (4 or 5)
Tissue (1)
Fine needle (not necessary for blackheads)
Book of matches or cigarette lighter

Blackheads

1. Your face is completely cleansed and exfoliated (see pages 85–86).
2. Sterilize blackhead remover (choose one of three methods, page 96).
3. Apply hot compress for five minutes (page 97).
4. Dab the pore to be treated with alcohol saturated cotton.
5. Looking into magnifying mirror, place smaller hole of blackhead remover on blackhead. Make sure you are on target.
6. Exert quick, firm pressure, ever so slightly to one side. If it did not release, try once more.
7. Upon release of matter, dab the pore with alcohol saturated cotton.
8. Clean out hole of extractor with twisted corner of tissue dipped in alcohol. Examine the matter (see page 97).
9. Proceed to the next blackhead (do not treat if less than ¼

inch away). Do not treat more than three blackheads, whiteheads, or pimples at any one session.

Upon examination, blackhead appears cone-shaped with narrow end being lighter in color. It is due to a plugged up sebaceous (oil) gland, otherwise it is a clog due to the environment. Do not wear foundation makeup and avoid moisturizer in that area for at least a day.

Whiteheads

Repeat all blackhead steps to point 4 above.

1. Sterilize tip of fine needle under match flame for a few seconds. Remove black carbon by wiping with alcohol-saturated cotton.
2. Dab whitehead with fresh cotton saturated in alcohol.
3. Look into magnifying mirror. Puncture the enclosed whitehead dead center.
4. Place smaller hole of blackhead remover on the whitehead, making sure you are on target.
5. Exert quick firm pressure ever so slightly to one side.
6. Then follow previously described blackhead steps starting at #7.

Upon examination, whiteheads appear as hard, round, waxy matter. Do not wear foundation makeup and avoid moisturizer in that area for at least a day.

Pimples

Follow instructions 1–3 in blackhead removal. In addition, instructions 1–3 in whitehead removal.

1. Place larger of the two holes dead center on pimple.
2. Upon release of matter, wipe area with alcohol saturated cotton.
3. Turn extractor over and use the smaller hole to release secondary matter. Wait another day to see if the entire impurity was

extracted. If not, give the skin a chance to recuperate and then repeat the procedure.

4. Dab the pore with alcohol saturated cotton.
5. Resume steps 8 and 9 in blackhead removal.

Upon examination, the extracted internal matter appears as pus mixed with oil and other impurities loosely held together. Do not wear foundation makeup and avoid moisturizer in that area for at least a day.

Alternative Method

Use medicated drying and peeling ointment (see page 98).

EYEBROWS: FRAMING YOUR EYES

Tweezing Your Eyebrows

In order to tweeze your eyebrows properly, your magnifying mirror is essential (see pages 16–17). You really have to be able to see clearly in order to grasp a tiny individual hair with your tweezers.

You have undoubtedly read or heard, "Tweeze one hair at a time only and remove it in the direction it grows." There is good reason for this. When an individual hair is grasped at its base and is pulled in the exact direction it grows, it will simply *slip* out of its follicle—without pain or irritation to the skin.

Use a good tweezer. A slant type is the easiest for most women to handle. An additional tweezer with a flat edge is also handy in some areas when a stubborn hair eludes you. If you need to wear glasses in order to tweeze, a curved type tweezer with a scissor handle is best. **Twissors** by **Kurlash** and another by **Revlon** are widely available.

Cleanse area to be tweezed with soap and water, then wipe the brow area with a cotton ball saturated in alcohol, (70 percent rubbing alcohol) wiping *against* the growth pattern. This cleans the base of each hair and makes it stand up for easy plucking. I know many women will shudder at the thought of using alcohol of this strength on their faces, thinking how drying it is, but that is only relevant when used constantly and excessively. The benefits you attain by using this alcohol, are:

   • Alcohol contains an antiseptic or antibacterial agent and your tweezer tips as well as the brow area should always be thoroughly wiped with it.
   • Alcohol removes the excess oil present on your skin which makes your tweezer slip.
   • Alcohol speeds up the whole tweezing process because you usually get the hair you want to pluck the first time and you are not causing irritation and redness by re-treating the same pore.

The tweezing process will run more smoothly and quickly and the *temporary* drying effect of the alcohol is counteracted with moisturizer as soon as you're finished.

Place a clean tissue in front of you and deposit each plucked hair on it as you remove it. Continual plucking with even tiny hairs caught in the tweezer tips will not facilitate the removal of the next hair and you will find yourself re-treating the same hair without success. This is what causes redness and irritation. A tweezer head is a precision instrument and cannot close properly if matter is still enclosed in its grip.

During the tweezing process, it will occasionally be necessary to wipe the tips of the tweezer on the tissue to clean off the tiny amount of oil and skin flakes it picks up. Even this tiny amount on your tweezer tips will not permit you satisfactory and efficient removal.

Creaming the brow area first and then immediately proceeding to tweeze is absolutely counterproductive to the tweezing process. The oil buildup (from the cream, as well as your own) is simply working against you and your tweezer. If you wish, you may cream the brow area first to soften it, but make sure to wipe it away with tissue and then with cotton saturated in alcohol.

The next step is eyebrow shaping. This is the one area of your face—in fact, the only feature—over which you have complete and total control to change its appearance for better or for worse. It can actually make or break your entire appearance.

Additional Notes
on Tweezing the Eyebrows

• If you really feel twinges of pain when you tweeze, then wrap an ice cube in a tissue or plastic bag just before you start to pluck. Put it on the fleshy areas under the brows. It will help to anesthetize these areas where most pain is felt.

• Tweezing should be done as often as necessary. There is no rule. Some women may have to retweeze every week to ten days. Others may have stubs long enough to grasp with a tweezer within a day or two. Just take care of them as they show up.

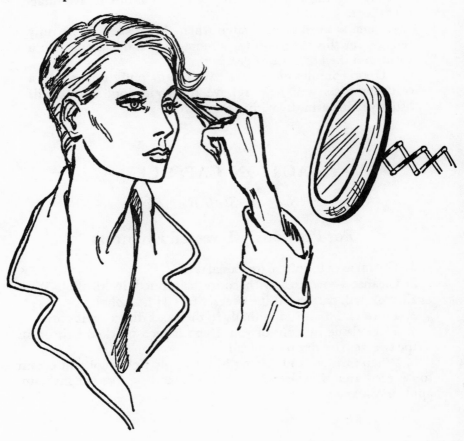

• The entire hair is removed including the hair bulb when you pluck it out in a straight pattern. If you do not have a firm grip on the base of the hair with your tweezers, it will break halfway down in the follicle, thereby growing back that much quicker. Since it takes time for the cells of the hair follicle to form and the papilla to nourish the resulting bulb from which the hair will grow out, obviously, you will have to tweeze less often.

• Tweezing or any other method of hair removal does not produce more hair or actually make the hairs thicker, stiffer, denser, or coarser. See page 111 regarding excess hair. If more hairs reappeared for every hair that was plucked, men would be tweezing the few hairs on their bald heads to manufacture more.

• Some women's eyes water when they tweeze. The only remedy for this is to stop for a moment and dry them with a tissue and then continue tweezing.

• Upon completion, if you have red or puffy upper lids, a cold compress will help relieve the condition, but it will usually fade naturally within the hour.

ACTION CAPSULE

(*Step-by-Step Review*)

For Previously Tweezed Eyebrows

1. Cream area to soften (optional).
2. Cleanse brow area with cotton saturated in alcohol. Wipe against growth pattern. Wipe tweezer tips with alcohol.
3. Pluck each hair individually in the exact direction it grows.
4. Place tissue in front of you. Deposit each plucked hair on it. Wipe tweezer tips dry periodically.
5. When finished and staying home, apply rich emollient cream to tweezed area. If going out, and/or intending to wear makeup, apply moisturizer.

Eyebrow Shaping

Determining where your eyebrows should start, peak, and end in relation to your eyes and the rest of your face is important and necessary. Your brows are one of the most expressive features you have, and all too often they do not conform to the rest of the face. Many natural facial expressions are often misinterpreted by other people because the brows do not reflect the real and natural you. Examine your own eyebrows. Try to analyze objectively if your brows express the real you. If not, you can either start from the beginning (previously unplucked eyebrows) or start all over again by allowing them to grow in, and then retweeze to give them a new and proper shape.

The "two pencil" method is the accepted technique for determining eyebrows' size and shape in the beauty business. But I like another method better because it's easier and more accurate. Take a piece of paper, fold it in half lengthwise. Continue to fold it lengthwise until it is about ½ inch wide. It is now flexible, has a definite edge, and you don't have to worry about paper cuts.

First, brush the brows in the direction they grow and then upward at the arch area so you can plainly see it. Hold the paper straight up, starting at the outside corner of the nostril and line it up with the inside corner of your eye. Any hairs appearing outside of the paper (toward the center of your face) should be removed.

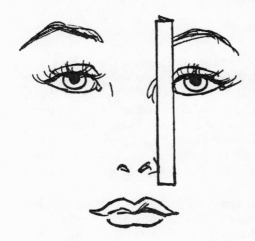

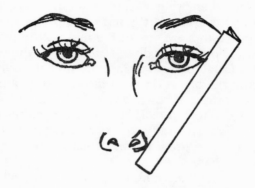

Don't get carried away and go further. Remove them hair by hair and recheck with the folded paper every so often.

Now, take the paper and line it up; again, starting at the corner of the nostril. (The paper fits nicely into the little tuck at the corner of the nostril.) Slant it toward the outside corner of your eye. Any excess hairs appearing past the upper edge of the paper should be tweezed out.

The Arch

Looking straight into the mirror, line the paper straight up on the outside of the iris (the colored portion of the eye), *not* the pupil (the small, dark center). This should be the highest point of the arch. Use an eyebrow brush to shape them into an upward curve. Remove just a few hairs from below the brow in order to accentuate the curve, then check to see if the arch is high enough. Don't overdo, but continue if you feel you need a higher arch. The higher the arch, the more it opens up the appearance of the eyes.

Now you are ready to remove all straggly hairs below the eyebrow. Leave the thickest area of hair on the inside next to nose and the thinnest part on the outside. Again, remove the hairs one by one and row by row. Repeat on the other eyebrow. Your aim is

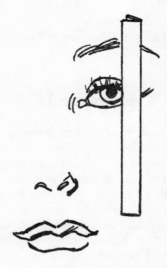

to get them as symmetrical as possible. No one ever gets this perfect because it is almost physically impossible, but your intention is to get them as much alike as you possibly can. If you find you have any excessively long hairs that are unruly but must remain as part of the brow, use a small scissors and clip only those hairs short enough to fit in with the rest.

It is a general rule not to pluck hairs above the eyebrows. But some rules must be broken for certain individuals. Don't pluck above the brows unless it is absolutely necessary; this can only be determined after you have shaped your eyebrows according to the above instructions. If there are still hairs above the browline that interfere with a good clean appearance, pluck them carefully and cautiously. You don't want to spend your life plucking away at your eyebrows!

Wipe the brows and the tips of the tweezers with alcohol. Then apply a rich, heavy cream to your brows to lubricate and soften them. This will allow your natural moisture to replenish itself.

The Nontweezer

When all is said and done, there are still some women who refuse to tweeze. This is fine for some, but for those women who have thick unruly brows, groom them daily with an eyebrow brush and use a bit of petroleum jelly (or mustache wax for very unruly hairs) to help hold a better line.

Eyebrows and Electrolysis

For the most part, I do not recommend electrolysis for eyebrows to shape them permanently. The exception to this rule is out-of-line hairs that would not be considered part of the brow line, or hairs so close to the eyelids that they close the eyes in.

Admittedly, this reasoning is long range in its approach. It is looking into the future when you are 70 or 80 years old. When there is sagging of skin and fine lines have become deep wrinkles. The contours of the face may then require reshaping of eyebrows to compensate and conform to the rest of the face. You can't do this if the hairs of your eyebrows are permanently removed. Therefore, you would have to totally rely on eyebrow pencil at a time of life when natural brows are more appealing and in keeping with old age. Remember too that eyebrow fashions change and thick eyebrows may again be revived long before you reach old age.

Eyebrow Coloring

Any great color contrast between eyebrows and hair is harsh and contributes to an aging appearance. Eyebrows should be in harmony with hair color—either the same color, as with redheads, or slightly darker, as with blondes and brownettes. Brunettes may want to go slightly lighter to alleviate any overall dark look. The general rule is to avoid marked contrasts and to achieve harmony for a natural appearance.

Bleaching and dyeing of eyebrows is a touchy and usually avoided subject, mainly because the Food and Drug Administration (FDA) does not permit manufacturers of hair dyes to instruct or encourage the consumer to use their products on eyebrows. While I know that many of you do this anyway and use them effectively and in reasonable safety, I must remind you that eyes are just too precious to threaten them with hair dye chemicals.

A beauty salon is the place to seek assistance, for their operators have the experience and control to attain just the right shade of eyebrows for your individual coloring.

ACTION CAPSULE

(Step-by-Step Review)

Eyebrow Shaping

1. Cream eyebrow area to soften for five minutes (optional). Remove with tissue and wipe only the area to be tweezed with alcohol-saturated cotton. Wipe against growth pattern. Also wipe tweezer tips.

2. Apply ice wrapped in tissue to fleshy areas (optional).

3. Fold paper lengthwise until ½ inch wide.

4. Brush brows in direction of growth.

5. Hold paper straight up between outside corner of nostril and inside corner of eye. Tweeze all hairs from bridge of nose to paper marking at corner of eye. Recheck with paper.

6. Make sure to pluck each hair in its direction of growth, and deposit on tisue. Wipe tweezer tips dry periodically.

7. Line paper up at corner of nostril to outside corner of eye. Tweeze hairs past upper edge of paper.

8. Line paper up on outside of colored iris for high point of arch. Brush into upward curve. Remove hairs cautiously, constantly rechecking your work.

9. Remove all straggly hairs below brow.

10. Repeat on other eyebrow.

11. Wipe brows and tweezer with cotton saturated alcohol.

12. Apply cream or moisturizer.

FACIAL HAIR

As we all advance in years, a small amount of facial hair may appear above the upper lip, on lower cheeks, and chin. It looks somewhat darker and sometimes feels coarser than normal facial hair. This is perfectly normal in anyone over 30 and its unsightliness can be easily remedied with bleach. For a more extreme solution, there is electrolysis for permanent removal of hair. There are two distinct types of electrolysis that will be discussed later.

For a not-too-serious case of a dark mustache above the lips, there are bleaching creams that are readily available and easy to use. **Andrea** and **Jolen** are two that are widely available. They are very effective, bleaching hair to an almost invisible blond in just a few minutes.

For that stubborn, occasional stiff hair or two you may find on your chin (please notice, I said one or two) pluck it out with a tweezer. It will grow back and you'll have to retweeze, but it won't encourage any new growth. *Caution:* If the hair is growing out of a mole, clip it short with a small scissors. Better yet, see your dermatologist to discuss possible mole removal.

A depilatory (chemical dissolver), for facial hair removal in cases of abundant peach fuzz (fine, light hair), will remove it temporarily at the surface level of the skin or slightly below. Admittedly one does become a slave to the removal of the ever-present regrowth. This should only be undertaken by women who will constantly keep it under control. A minimal or even a nominal amount of peach fuzz should not be considered for removal. But in some cases where it is truly abundant, removal is absolutely necessary for appearance's sake, as well as the well-being of the individual—but only on normal skin. Never use a depilatory on abraded, irritated, or sunburned skin. Aerosol depilatories are definitely dangerous as they might accidentally get into the eyes. Always use a patch test to determine in advance any allergic reaction to this type of product, particularly because its incidence is more prone on the face.

Waxing as a method of removing excessive hair, even peach fuzz, should be done by a professional. Beauty salons offer this service. This type of hair removal is very tricky, besides being quite painful when one applies it at home. However, it has the advantage of lasting for three to six weeks.

Women who are inclined toward dark coarse hair on the face should be cautious about removing it at all with either depilatory or wax methods. You should judge by previous experience with other body hair, such as on the legs or underarms. If the rate of growth is slow and the hair's regrowth is on the fine side, then you are a possible candidate. If the rate of growth is fast and the hair is rather coarse, you will be subject to a brittle, almost daily, 5 o'clock shadow that could be more disconcerting than the dark hair itself. In that case, you are better advised to use bleach.

The removal of hair has nothing to do with how fine or thick it will be when it regrows or, for that matter, its rate of growth. It is not the methods we use to remove hair—depilatory, wax, or shaving (which I don't recommend)—that make hair darker and coarser. The hair lacks the filament (which gives it flexibility) at the stage when it reappears just above the surface of the skin. This is what makes it appear coarse and feel stiff. In addition, the hair follicles then have a secure grip and are holding each individual hair very tightly in place. If allowed to grow out, the hairs will resume the characteristics they originally bore. By the same token, removal of hair will not produce more hair than had grown originally. The state of regrowth is completely dependent upon your internal metabolism.

When a slightly hairier appearance is first noticed, some women think it is due to certain creams they may have used. This is an old wives' tale! There is no external cream, lotion, ointment, or anything else that can grow hair. If there were, we would have no bald men in our society.

We all know from the experience of shaving our legs, that as the hair regrows the short shafts that appear above the skin surface are stiff, for the reasons explained above. This stubble appears coarse and the feel of it is undesirable and even offensive. So while it may be necessary to employ one of the above removal measures for your face, I caution you to examine the matter very carefully before employing it. If you think the hair on your face is getting just a little too excessive, then medical advice should be sought. The growth rate and the kind of hair produced are controlled primarily by hormones produced by the ovaries, adrenal, and pituitary glands. A thorough examination by your doctor may disclose an underlying cause for the excess hair problem and result in a solution.

More than half of the women in this country experience excess facial hair following menopause. This is due to hormonal changes that normally take place as a result of menopause. Your physician should be consulted concerning problems of excess hair.

Hirsutism is abnormal, excessive hair, which, when it appears on the face, is abundant, coarse, dark, and thick. This form of excessive hair may be caused by severe hormone imbalance or other physical dysfunction. A consultation with your physician is definitely in order, through which it may be corrected.

Up to now we have been talking about relatively minor quantities of facial hair and how to deal with the problem on a temporary basis. We will assume in the more extreme cases that you are checked by a physician to see that there are no underlying medical causes.

Now we come to a point where a form of permanent hair removal should be considered for both the mild and more extreme cases. This is not as costly as one might think, especially when viewed in terms of the convenience and the ultimate pleasure it will provide.

Permanent Hair Removal

Electrolysis is the long-time method of permanent removal of hairs, one by one. The procedure involves a very fine needle being inserted into each hair follicle, and delivering an electric current to destroy the papilla that nourishes the hair bulb from which the hair grows out. The process is relatively painless but one should put oneself into the hands of a very competent professional for this method. Otherwise, scarring and pitting can occur.

There is also a new method to permanently remove hair that has now stood the test of time and therefore can be recommended. It is called Depilatron. This is an electronic unit connected to a special type of tweezer that plucks out the hairs, one by one, while simultaneously sending a non-painful electric current down the hair shaft to destroy its papilla. Depilatron is fast and removes even stubborn curly hairs in a much shorter period of time than necessary for electrolysis. There is no risk of pitting or scarring because nothing is inserted into the hair follicle, nor does it touch the surface of the skin.

There are many Depilatron technicians operating in beauty salons throughout the country. And because the process is so easy and relatively inexpensive, there are bound to be many more in the not too distant future. Let's face it . . . women just don't like excess hair regardless of its quantity anywhere on their bodies, much less their faces.

Summing Up:

The likely candidates for permanent hair removal where the expense is affordable are:
* The woman with a slightly dark mustache that needs periodic bleaching.
* The woman with a dark, coarse mustache that bleaches, waxes, or uses a depilatory.
* The woman with a few scattered strong, stiff hairs, that she is plucking out or clipping close to the skin.
* The woman who has curly hairs which tend to become ingrown causing blemishes.
* The woman with slight to medium growth of dark coarse hair on the lower cheeks. (Medium and heavier growth should be checked by a physician first.)
* Post-menopausal women after consulting physician.
* The woman who has a closed-in forehead where removal of selective hairs would open up and give better balance to the face.
* Women who have thick dark hairs over their nose and between eyebrows. Caution: do not permanently remove any hairs beyond the inner corners of the eyes.

Candidates for permanent hair removal where the expenditure is more sizable and time consuming. Warning: Consult a physician first for possible underlying causes.
* Women who have more than a medium amount of hair on the lower cheeks.
* Women who are considered hirsute.

FACIAL EXERCISE

The only known cure for droopy eyelids or loose skin anywhere on the face or neck is cosmetic surgery. Facial massage and exercise—not to be confused with body massage or exercise—have long been debated with experts never agreeing whether it is helpful or harmful.

My theory is: when in doubt—do nothing! However, if this is something you feel has worked for you in the past, and you are personally satisfied, then by all means, do not let me dissuade you. Please, just don't recommend it to your friends (if you really like them). The outcome is still controversial and may accelerate the aging process or create permanent damage. If you understand the stress and strain that is put upon the collagen and elastic fibers described on page 29, then you must understand that facial exercise is more than likely injurious to the face and be opposed to the practice. What is good for the body is not necessarily good for the head. The two must be regarded separately if for no other reason than that facial muscles are directly attached to the skin. This is totally opposite to that of the body, where every muscle is attached to bone. Because of this, it is highly conceivable that if facial muscles were never used, sagging and wrinkling would never occur.

NECK EXERCISE

For cosmetic purposes, the neck is always considered part of the face, but when it comes to exercise we have to make a departure and classify the neck again with the body. Exercising to tone the muscles of the body and to stay in shape is high on everyone's stay-healthy list. There are no disputes when it comes to exercising the body, except perhaps which exercises are best for each individual. Exercising the muscles of the neck is also a good idea, but it becomes a bad one when deliberate contortions of the face are linked to the motions used in certain neck exercises. (And more often than not, this is the case.) Here is a simple exercise to tone the muscles of the neck that you can integrate with your other exercises.

1. Let your head hang off the edge of the bed and slowly bring it to a parallel position with your body.

2. Then slowly lower it again.

3. Repeat ten times, counting each time you raise your head.

OLD STANDBYS: "FROWNIES," CHIN STRAPS AND HEADBANDS

There are a couple of external devices that are worth mentioning here. They were widely used in "the good ole days" but passed out of vogue some time back. I think these are worth resurrecting for some women under certain circumstances. I am referring to "frownies" and chin straps. Indeed, these are not cure-alls or preventatives. They merely help by retarding or minimizing an already existing facial tendency.

The woman who has a tendency toward a deep frown line between her eyebrows (medically known as *glabella*) should know that it does not respond particularly well to cosmetic surgery, since surgery can only soften the line. This line appears to be more pronounced with time, but a frownie will help the groove from becoming more accentuated. A frownie is a small patch with an adhesive backing worn at night and perhaps around the house. They might be difficult to find but are available through mail-order houses. (Check in the back section of almost any women's magazine.) There is one precaution that needs to be emphasized, which is to remove the frownie with extremely gentle care.

For the woman whose jawline is becoming more noticebly dropped with the natural pull of gravity, and in certain situations such as reading in bed which tends to accelerate the tendency with even further pull . . . a chin strap will help to hold back the sagging. (Also, more readily available through mail-order houses.)

For either of these devices to help, their consistent use is imperative. Best results are obtained by wearing them nightly when the skin and facial muscles are more relaxed, and, of course, night also presents the most convenient time. However, one must use her discretion. One certainly doesn't appear very sexy wearing these contraptions in front of her man. (That's probably the reason they passed out of vogue in the first place.)

When in public view there is still another external appliance to be considered. Headband devices that provide a temporary face lift have been used by theatrical people for some time. I think they are only appropriate for the mature average woman for special occasions. The bands work on the chin line tightening the sagging skin of the lower half of the face. The final aesthetic effect depends upon how much lifting a woman needs, although there is always some improvement. Many women who are inclined to use these devices usually have a tendency to wear them too tightly, causing headaches. Other than this they are not supposedly harmful to an already sagging skin, although too frequent wearing could prove otherwise. They are made of elastic bands or cords that are tied around the head and attached at the temples with special glue or adhesive tape which must then be concealed by makeup and a camouflaging hairstyle or wig.

While these devices are also available through mail-order houses, I think it is prudent to purchase them where one can get the "feel" of them and where trained help can be sought, since proper fit and application are crucial for appearance and comfort.

COSMETIC SURGERY

There comes a time in a woman's life, usually in the late 40s or early 50s, when she looks in the mirror and is distressed by what she sees. This may occur even earlier if she has been a sun worshiper, but the moment of truth is considerably delayed if she has adhered to a good care and maintenance regimen. Nonetheless, the despondency she feels can be especially acute if she has been a woman who, up to this time, has possessed a certain air of self-confidence sprinkled with a healthy amount of vanity. The wrinkles, deep furrows, and sagging of skin that stare back at her from the mirror give cause for her to wonder if she should consider a face lift. And if so, is she being unduly vain? There are other women who arrive at this stage of life and their mirrors reflect a different kind of self-confidence. This one says, "I've earned every one of those wrinkles and I'll wear them proudly!" Both attitudes are right! My philosophy concerning this and all other situations in life is: Every woman should do what is right for herself as long as she doesn't hurt or deprive anyone else. Attitude is the important factor here, rather than the specifics of surgical techniques. For anyone who requires that kind of data, there are several very good books dealing solely with cosmetic plastic surgery, and I highly recommend them when the question,

"Should I, or shouldn't I?" becomes more than a fleeting thought. (Besides the surgical techniques, these books discuss costs, indica- tions, contra-indications, physical discomfort, fears, anxieties, and just about any question that initially comes to mind plus a great deal more.) *

If a woman feels that her improved physical appearance will spark her interests in the outside world, give her renewed vitality, and generally lift her spirits, then by all means she is a good can- didate. Cosmetic facial surgeons will not accept everyone, in par- ticular the woman who wants the surgery for what they consider the wrong motives, which might be any psychological problem deemed out of proportion. Fortunately, most women are realistic (about 90 percent) and are good candidates.

A face lift (*rhytidectomy*) will rejuvenate the person who has it by five to ten years but will not cause a halt to the aging process. The lift is also expected to last five to ten years after which sub- sequent lifts are usually necessary. There doesn't seem to be any definite maximum number of operations one may undergo—it de- pends upon the individual. Certain actresses are reputed to have had many. But there is good reason for this as their profession con- stantly calls for using facial muscles and various contortions of the face, not normally used by others, in order to act out their scenes and make their dramatic points. (Another reason to support the theory that facial exercise, undue manipulation, and deep massage cause premature aging. It's called *overuse!*)

Some women complain of extra folds in their eyelids and there- fore find it difficult to use eye makeup. Even though they would like to wear it they feel they must avoid its use. Eyelid surgery (*blepharoplasty*) to correct the superfluous skin of the eyelids

---

* *Doctor, Make Me Beautiful*, James W. Smith, M.D. (David McKay Co.) 1973.

Consultation with a Plastic Surgeon, Ralph Leslie Dicker, M.D. and Victor Royce Syracuse, M.D. (Nelson Hall) 1975.

Plastic Surgery: Beauty You Can Buy, Harriet La Barre (Holt, Rinehart and Winston) 1970.

The Miracle of Cosmetic Plastic Surgery, Richard B. Aronsohn, M.D. and Richard A. Epstein, Ph.D. (Sherbourne Press, Inc.) 1970.

A New You, James O. Stallings, M.D., with Terry Morris (Mason/Charter) 1977.

Cosmetic Surgery: A Consumer's Guide, Sylvia Rosenthal (Tree Lippin- cott) 1977.

and/or around the eyes is very gratifying to the woman who has
these problems. (This is quite prevalent in even younger age
groups, heredity being the main factor causing this condition.)
This surgery, although extremely delicate and requiring painstak-
ing skill on the part of the surgeon, is the most rewarding in terms
of restoring a youthful look to the entire face. It is also known to
have a brief recovery period, the most predictable outcome of all
cosmetic surgery, and lasts from ten to fifteen years. Neck lifts and
restoring the jowls and lower jaw to a firm, more youthful outline
are also said to be extremely gratifying to the woman who feels she
has aged virtually overnight. Of course, this is also performed as
part of the standard face lift.

Let's go back to, "Should I or shouldn't I?" If any of these signs
of aging or inherited anomalies makes you feel unhappy with
yourself and you simply want to look better, with a few years
erased from your face, and if you do not feel intimidated by anyone else but truly want it for your own emotional and physical
well-being, then of course, you should consult a reputable cosmetic plastic surgeon. Not one, but two or three. It is far wiser to
spend extra money for consultation fees to determine which doctor you best relate to (communications are important), and who
will fulfill your expectations (because no two surgeons work exactly alike) , than to regret later your hasty decision of the first
doctor. And don't be afraid to ask questions of the doctor or ask
to meet his patients who have had similar surgery, to determine
the aesthetic effects for yourself. (If you are shy or have second
thoughts concerning the latter, bear in mind that it is not an un-
usual request and is sometimes welcomed. The doctor you are consulting may or may not see fit to do so but you have the right
to ask.)

The local office of your county medical society will supply you
with a list of names in your area that you can investigate. Or your
local library most likely has a copy of the *Directory of Medical
Specialists* which lists board certified doctors in all branches of
medicine under the auspices of the American Medical Association
(AMA) . Or, you can write to the American Society of Plastic and
Reconstructive Surgeons, Inc., 29 East Madison Street, Chicago,
Illinois 60602. In Canada contact the Royal College of Physicians
and Surgeons of Canada, 74 Stanley Street, Ottawa, Ontario. Most

countries throughout the world have their equivalent of these professional associations. Always ask for the names of at least three plastic surgeons who specialize in *cosmetic or aesthetic surgery*. And remember that your own physician can also refer several cosmetic plastic surgeons. Then, let thoughtful, intelligent decision-making be your guide.

All of the cleansing and makeup procedures outlined in this book are approved by cosmetic plastic surgeons. Nonetheless, you should double check with *your* doctor to make sure *he* approves. Cosmetic surgeons generally agree that complete makeup may be used two weeks after surgery. Most women who have undergone cosmetic surgery feel they require new makeup and seek out new techniques. Many go to special classes exclusively for this purpose. You may be sure that the makeup techniques that follow shortly are designed for you after surgery as well as before. The techniques are very much the same as those taught in special classes.

As I mentioned before, there are women who will wear their wrinkles proudly and they *should* do just that! They should not feel intimidated or bear the brunt of criticism because their peers (and this is descriptive of certain social circles) say, "At our age, cosmetic surgery is the thing to do." If you are secure and content with who you are, what you are, and how you look, pay no heed to what the girls say. You are your own individual!

Major Facial Flaws

Keloids are claw-like fibrous overgrowths of scar tissue and can be successfully removed by plastic surgery even though there is some risk of the scar reoccurring. It is up to the plastic surgeon to determine who is and who is not a good candidate. The procedure followed here usually involves trading a serious, thickly raised scar for a fine, flat, smaller scar which in some cases can be hidden in the natural folds of the skin. On the other hand, some keloids can be treated by a dermatologist with injected medication which causes the keloid tissue to shrink. X-ray therapy is sometimes indicated (and is prescribed for the body) but is discouraged on most areas of the face. These are all problems to be solved by the chosen doctor and it is certainly worth investigating if you have keloids or are prone to them.

Black and oriental women have a high incidence of keloids mainly due to the fact that there is a greater concentration of melanin in their skin. In areas devoid of melanin such as the palms of hands and soles of feet, keloids do not occur. Among Caucasians, keloids are largely due to genetic influences and even very fair blonde women can be predisposed to the condition.

Minor Facial Flaws

Broken capillaries (red, spidery lines), moles, warts, brown liver spots, skin tags, and other small blemishes can all be treated in a dermatologist's office.

The doctor merely touches a broken capillary with an electric needle which fuses the walls of the tiny red web thereby eliminating the flow of blood through them which gives the spot its red appearance. This process feels like no more than a little prick of the skin with a momentary burning sensation so it doesn't even require an anesthetic.

Moles that are well placed are sometimes a beauty asset. If not, some kinds of moles can be removed with the electric needle, causing them to dry up. Other types of moles need to be surgically removed. In this case, the incidence of a tiny scar from the operation depends upon the individual. Of course, many women are not bothered by moles regardless of where they occur, but the moles should always be checked for possible malignancy.

Warts, on the other hand, should be removed as soon as they appear. Warts are caused by a virus and can easily spread, causing more warts. The longer you let them go the more they multiply and the more likely that scarring will take place when you do have them removed. The electric needle here also is the instrument that the dermatologist usually uses to rid them quickly and safely, with only momentary minor pain.

Small brown spots commonly called liver spots or age spots are also aided by a minor treatment in the dermatologist's office. As in the treatment of broken capillaries, he treats them with the electric needle, or he may use cryosurgery. This is a method that freezes the spot, causing it to blister which results in fresh new skin. Or he may use another method that he feels is more suitable to the particular condition. I've heard so many women say, "If only I could get rid of these horrible, brown spots." (Bleaching creams more often than not are ineffective.) They don't know that the dermatologist has an answer to their lament.

Skin tags and other small blemishes are also dispatched usually with the electric needle or cryosurgery.

Dermabrasion and Chemical Face Peels

Dermabrasion—skin planing that uses a small, high-speed revolving wire brush, diamond fraise, or sanding disk—and chemical face peels—*chemabrasion* (light peel) or *chemosurgery* (deep peel)—are methods to improve the quality of skin. They can offer a new lease on life for those women who suffer from acne scars, and in some cases the condition of active acne can be improved. Other candidates for these techniques are those who want to rid themselves of vertical lines above the upper lip, or they have lesions, raised scars, flat warts, brown liver spots, or certain types of moles, even freckles. Additionally, *dermabrasion* and/or *chemosurgery* are sometimes used in conjunction with cosmetic plastic surgery (but usually not at the same time), to refine the texture of skin, improve smoothness by erasing fine, imbedded wrinkles, and reducing the depth of other wrinkles. Even though the patient is adequately medicated and anesthetized, one must have a fair tolerance for pain to undergo these procedures, and also necessary are realistic expectations which the doctor will explain beforehand. All of these methods (including *chemabrasion*) which remove the outer layers of the epidermis in order for new skin to replace itself, are areas of medicine that should only be practiced by highly skilled, extremely qualified cosmetic plastic surgeons or dermatologists. There are many lay people also practicing these techniques who inflict tragic, horrible results on an unsuspecting public. I cannot emphasize strongly enough the vital responsibility on the part of a prospective patient to consult a fully accredited, licensed doctor and not a so-called specialist whose only degree is in cosmetology and not in medicine. A reliable cosmetologist will never attempt more than a "mini-peel" which does not involve the strong chemicals used in *chemabrasion* and *chemosurgery*.

Silicone

The word silicone itself causes understandable confusion, and requires the sorting out of its benefits and contraindications. Silicone implants of a solid, pure grade medical variety are commonly used in plastic surgery to attain certain physical characteristics such as the augmentation of a receding chin (*mentoplasty*). This is accepted medical practice and has been for more than twenty-five years. This kind of silicone and the techniques employed for its implantation are quite different from liquid silicone injections which are used to puff out wrinkles, to plump up deep frown lines between the eyebrows, or elevate the nasolabial lines between nose and mouth.

Liquid silicone injections are still in the experimental stages because they reportedly stray from the injected site. In the late 1960s and early 1970s, small injections of liquid silicone held considerable promise for the medical profession. The highly publicized huge amounts that were injected into the breasts of chorus girls are a different story. At this writing there are only eight doctors in the entire United States who are licensed by the Food and Drug Administration (FDA) to use liquid silicone experimentally for injection purposes only. Experimentation has been going on since 1965. Only these eight doctors have access to pure, sterile, unadulterated special, medical-grade liquid silicone which is tightly controlled by its manufacturer, Dow Corning Corporation, and the FDA. Unless you are extremely venturesome, don't seek to be a guinea pig—the real thing just isn't available. If and when this special medical-grade silicone moves out of its clinical investigation phase and is FDA approved, then it will be in widespread use. At that time, you might consider it.

Fibrin Foam Technique

The fibrin foam technique now holds much promise for those women with deep pitted, irregular, or wavelike acne scars. This is a relatively new technique and it is no longer in the experimental stages.

The technique involves utilizing one's own blood. The dermatologist draws enough to fill a small-size test tube. It is performed as an office procedure and you are asked to return to the office in about a week. In the meantime, the blood is processed by a laboratory which extracts the blood protein (*fibrin,* a chemical constituent of blood clots). It is used to treat the scar by injection with a very small needle just below the surface of the skin to fill in and puff up even deep craters permanently. Since your own blood is used there is no problem of rejection. The fibrin foam technique is reported to be quick, safe, relatively inexpensive as compared to other methods, and virtually painless.

If you have any type of depressed scar and you are interested in this treatment, consult your dermatologist, the dermatology department of your local hospital, or a university-affiliated medical center who will refer you to a dermatologist who uses this technique. However, I must caution you: Not all dermatologists will be enthusiastic, and this new treatment, too, is bound to have its adversaries. As with any new medical treatment, a major concern is the long-term effect, and only the test of time is the ultimate truth. Let's hope that this one is here to stay.

ALLERGIES

Be fair to yourself and to the products you buy. Many women with very slight knowledge make the assumption that they are allergic to a product. They might simply have eaten something that day which caused the allergic reaction. The circumstantial evidence then costs the women money, for in all likelihood that makeup is thrown away or never used again. Other women say that they are allergic to a whole line of products just because they don't happen to like the brand name. No kidding, I've run across this many times.

Naturally, you must like the product in order for it to make you feel good, before it can even make you look good, but "I'm allergic to that" is a much overplayed comment. Be sure, it's your money! However, if you do have an existing or ongoing problem consult a dermatologist.

Labeling

It is now mandated by law that the ingredients of all cosmetics and toiletries (perfumes and soaps excluded) be listed in descending order of quantity on the label of every product. If the label is too small, then it must be accompanied by an attached tag. (If this listing is omitted in either form, it is an indication that the product is old.) The cosmetic and toiletry industries fought this compulsory listing for many years, arguing that it was of no value to the consumer and only provided easy access for competitors to duplicate or steal formulas. This seemingly jaundiced view does have merit because where the consumer is concerned she would need a degree in biochemistry to comprehend the many highly technical terms that comprise the listing. (Cosmetic dictionaries also help the consumer.) However, labeling has at least one immediate practical purpose. That is that one can check the label for ingredients that are known to cause allergic reactions. Of course your dermatologist or physician must make you aware of them. However, with time you may be able to determine some specific allergic reactions for yourself as we shall see.

Patch Test for Allergic Reaction

There is a very simple test that you can give to yourself to see if any* given product will produce an allergic reaction. And it is possible to develop such a reaction even after years of using one's favorite product.

You simply apply a generous portion of the product in question, full strength, to a small area of the inner surface of the forearm and place an adhesive bandage over it. Check after 24 hours to see if there is any redness, swelling, or blistering. If none, leave the bandage in place and check again in another 24 hours. If after 48 hours there is no skin reaction, then you can be assured that you are not allergic to that product.

If the skin shows a slight redness, you have some sensitivity to the product and its use should be discontinued. Anything more,

---

* Lipstick, mascara, eyeliner, eyeshadow, concealer, highlighter, foundation, blush or rouge, sunscreen/sunblock, creams and lotions.

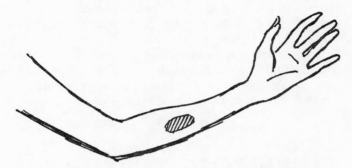

Apply here and cover with adhesive bandage.

such as blistering or swelling, means you are allergic and you should stop using that particular brand of cosmetic and switch to another, first checking the label to compare the main ingredients and make sure that they are not duplicated. I must caution you, however, not to jump to conclusions. This aspect of the test is a time consuming task that requires isolating a specific ingredient only by process of elimination.

Hypo-Allergenic Cosmetics

Hypo-allergenic is a term applied to two distinct areas of cosmetic manufacture.

The first type includes cosmetics that are "fragrance free" (containing no perfume) and are manufactured, filled, and packaged under continually monitored and highly controlled conditions. It is a fact that *half* the known allergies affecting the allergy-prone person are found in fragrances. It is also a fact that almost every cosmetic of every reputable established manufacturer's line is compounded and packaged under the same safeguarded conditions.

The second type includes cosmetics which entirely eliminate ingredients *known* to cause allergy. Almay, Ar-Ex, and Marcelle are three cosmetic brands which are manufactured to this standard that dermatologists recognize and endorse. For years these companies supplied the dermatologist with a report of their own individual lines, listing every ingredient in every product for their reference so that they could more readily isolate a specific ingredient. Of course now listing of all ingredients in cosmetics is mandatory.

Most women are not as susceptible to allergy as they might think. But if you do experience such a reaction, see your dermatologist or use the patch test on the preceding page before discarding the product. You may be throwing out good money.

COMMERCIAL VS. HOMEMADE PRODUCTS

Commercial cosmetics do not require refrigeration, as they have built-in safe-guards that natural homemade cosmetics using fruits, vegetables, dairy products, plant extracts, etc., cannot provide.* The homemade variety must be refrigerated to prevent spoilage, and refrigeration in itself offers a limited shelf life. The word "preservative" bears a disagreeable connotation in today's society, but one must remember that cosmetic preservatives are not ingested. Besides preventing spoilage, preservatives in cosmetic products are a necessary element to fight germs and are extremely effective in controlling micro-organisms and contamination that would otherwise spread infection or disease.** Every time you open and close a homemade, natural, or commercial product, applying it to yourself from its container, there is the risk of contamination because micro-organisms exist everywhere. The minute but effective quantities of preservatives contained in commercial cosmetic products act as a sterilizer so that you are assured of safe usage over a considerable period of time.

If you have the time and patience to mix a fresh batch of product every time you need it, then by all means it is safe (provided you are not allergic to it). If you have any left over, be sure to refrigerate it and use it quickly.

---

* In hot climates, where the product would melt, refrigeration is advisable.
** So called "natural" or "organic" cosmetics sold over the counter also require preservatives, otherwise they are subject to the same shortcomings of the homemade variety.

PART II
MAKEUP

Makeup!
The Excitement
Begins

Yesterday, the whole fashion trend encouraged loss of identity. Today, we are individuals doing our own things. But it is up to you, and you only, to bring out the best individual woman that is within you. A bland picture of personal tidiness is not enough— there is more to you and you can be more beautiful!

With the newly improved, more radiant skin which is about to be yours because you now know how to care for and manage it (using the proper cleansing procedures, including exfoliation and moisturizers) , the world of makeup is at your doorstep.

There is no one correct way to do *anything!* The instructions and procedures I outline are by no means the only ones. They are just the easiest ways to bring out the best and most beautiful, individual you. They are universally accepted by all experts in this field. Of course, they may also have other or additional ideas. Where there is opinion there will always be dispute, but this is minor dispute among experts. Another case entirely, and one that gets my temper up and makes me see red, is a current beauty who is riding the crest of popularity, with publicity in the media, trying to impose her *personal* routine and advice—as if it were gospel—on millions of unsuspecting women. The information she hands out is usually incorrect, often antiproductive, and in some cases downright destructive. Her personal regimen may work for her but she is without background, foundation, and knowledge as to what happens to millions of other women who may think she knows all.

Some makeup experts might recommend putting an under eye concealer on *after* your tinted foundation. I call for application after moisturizer and *before* foundation, and I give you my reasons why. Common sense provides your best solution. No one procedure is absolutely right for everyone and it is up to you to alter, but not depart from the routine.

Taking Care of Your Looks Is Great for Your Morale!

This is makeup to be yourself—to fulfill your potential as an individual woman—not to transform you, just to be your best. While imitation of another woman may be the sincerest form of flattery, simulation of that woman is the pinnacle of self-deceit. Be true to yourself and your individual type. Be pretty for yourself first, and then you will be pretty for all eyes that fall upon you.

Many women apply makeup for daytime as if they were going to a glamorous gala affair. This tendency to overdo is pathetically cruel to the total effect. In most cases, it is the result of a heavy hand, and a little restraint is all that is called for.

You need awareness, but you also need follow-through. And you must be cognizant of the fact that something new does not always seem right at first. In all fairness to yourself, you should give any new idea or technique at least a three-day trial before you discard it.

The Mystery of Night

Evening makeup is really not much more than the application of more vivid colors, including frosteds and luminescents for more sparkle under night lights, when daytime makeup would fade. However, the main difference between daytime and nighttime makeup is a slightly heavier application. It is always preferable to start fresh to make up for the evening. However, in instances when one does not have the time for a complete re-do, all that is really required to meet the challenge of the evening is to freshen up the complexion by adding more blush or rouge, to change the lipstick shade, and to apply more vivid colors to the eyes, with a heavier application of mascara either with or without false eyelashes.

WHO MAKES THE BEST MAKEUP?

The Food and Drug Administration (FDA) states: "Federal law—the Food, Drug and Cosmetic Act—does not require that a cosmetic fulfill all the hopes and dreams that may be encouraged by its advertising."

Over the years, the one question most frequently asked of me by countless women is, "What cosmetic company makes the best makeup?" To this, I have a stock but truthful reply, "It's not what you use but how you use it!" The words are accurate but, of course, all too brief. No one could be more aware than I that the answer is inadequate. However, it seems to answer that burning question for the moment since the reaction is almost always a self-assured, "Well I always knew it! Now what do I do?" These pages afford me the opportunity to expand on those oft-repeated words.

All established cosmetic companies are reputable and they all produce good cosmetic products—they are all safe and this is especially so today. If not, they are quickly recalled by the manufacturer. There have been very few deleterious products that have slipped out onto the retail cosmetic shelf. It's just too expensive for any manufacturer to make this kind of mistake. You can be sure that each and every product by every established manufacturer is thoroughly tested on hundreds (sometimes thousands) of users before it is marketed. And not only each and every product, but every color within that product line. I know, I speak firsthand! As a former product development and marketing manager, this was one of my most important areas of concern.

Color products vary from manufacturer to manufacturer. The same product type used for the same purpose may be available as a cream, gel, liquid, or powder. They vary in texture, both look and feel. And, there are various consistencies from sheer to opaque, but they are all good. It is how you use them that makes the vital difference on your face. As a former director of beauty techniques, I could take the most inexpensive color cosmetics and achieve the same results on a model that I could with the most expensive brands. I have worked for cosmetic companies from the low end to the highest of the economic spectrum, and many in-between.

While many cosmetic companies try to promote brand loyalty among their customers, it is certainly possible to use, for example, a rather expensive tinted foundation (because you like the shade and texture and perhaps even the perfume it contains), an eyebrow pencil or mascara from an inexpensive company (because you like the shade of pencil or think the consistency is just right for your lashes), and a blusher or lipstick from yet another company because you like the color and glow.

I do not say this in order to confuse you, but rather because many women have the idea that color cosmetics from only one company will go together harmoniously. This simply is not the case. It is knowing which types of products go together that produces the end result—your radiant look. It is not only possible, but more than likely, that you could wear every single type of cosmetic and still look more natural than the woman who only wears blue eyeshadow and pink lipstick.

All cosmetics are based on the type of tinted foundation you use and whether or not you use face powder. There are only two types of tinted foundation to consider after the age of 30—liquid or cream. There is only one type of face powder to consider and is referred to as either translucent or transparent. (See pages 180 and 182 regarding tinted face powders.)

The following is a list of the types of products to be used with either liquid or cream foundation, taking into account whether or not you use face powder. Products are listed in order of application on the face.

HOW TO PUT DIFFERENT TYPE PRODUCTS TOGETHER

LIQUID FOUNDATION (BASE)

Moisturizer—correlated to skin type

Under eye concealer—cream, gel, or swivel stick

Tinted liquid foundation (base)

Blush or rouge—If using face powder afterwards, cream, gel, crayon, or liquid; If not using face powder, dry or powdered type

Translucent or transparent face powder

Eyebrow pencil—If using before face powder, crayon type; If using after face powder, cake or powdered type; If not using face powder, powdered or cake type

Eyeshadow—If using before face powder, gel, liquid, or crayon; If using after face powder, crayon, cream, swivel stick, or cake or powdered type; If using no powder, any type

Eyeliner—any type: liquid, pencil, cake, or automatic applicator

Mascara—Any type: cream, cake, or automatic applicator

CREAM FOUNDATION (BASE)

Moisturizer—correlated to skin type

Under eye concealer—cream, gel, semi-liquid, or swivel stick

Tinted cream foundation (base)

Blush or rouge—If using face powder afterwards, cream, crayon, or stick form; If not using face powder, dry or powdered type

Translucent or transparent face powder

Eyebrow pencil—If using before face powder, crayon type; If using after face powder, cake or powdered type; If not using face powder, cake or powdered type

Eyeshadow—If using before face powder, gel, cream, crayon, or swivel stick; If using after face powder, crayon, powdered, or cake type; If using no face powder, any type

Eyeliner—Any type: liquid, pencil, cake, or automatic applicator

Mascara—Any type; cream, cake, or automatic applicator

LIQUID FOUNDATION (BASE)

Lipstick—If using face powder before, any type; If using no face powder, one that is not too creamy or lip gloss by itself; A gloss may be used over any lipstick (do not blot any lipstick)

CREAM FOUNDATION (BASE)

Lipstick—If using face powder before, any type; If using no face powder, one that is not too creamy or gloss by itself; A gloss may be used over any lipstick (do not blot any lipstick)

BALANCE AND HARMONY

Play Up Your Best Features and Bring Other Features Into Balance

Few women have a clear picture of themselves as they really are. After a complete cleansing, when your face is nude as nude can be, take a good long objective look at your face in the mirror. Be highly critical. Decide if your skin tone needs perking up or toning down (see page 136). Decide if your eyebrows are properly suited to your eyes and to your face as a whole (see page 105). Determine the shape of your face (see pages 151–157) and decide if you need a slight bit of contouring and/or a new hairstyle (see page 150). Hairstyles play a big part in accenting and correcting the shape of a face. Study your face. Judge which are your best features—eyes, nose, or mouth.

To determine whether your eyes are closely spaced or widely spaced, project the width of one of your eyes to the distance between both of your eyes. You can do this by measuring with a piece of paper and marking it. If the distance is equal, your eyes are evenly spaced. If less or more, you can bring them into better alignment with eye makeup.

If your eyes and nose are large, then play up your mouth with bright shades of lipstick. Diminish the size of the nose with a slight bit of contour shading to bring everything into proportion.

If your eyes are small or deep set, your nose medium size, and your mouth large, then concentrate on your eyes and stay inside

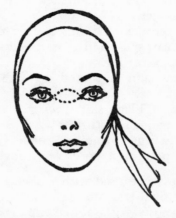

your lipline with your lipstick, using a lipbrush, crayon, or pencil made for this purpose.

If your nose is large, your eyes small and your mouth medium size, then heavier emphasis (not to be confused with heavier eye makeup) is put on the eyes to bring them into proportion. The nose, which in this case seems to overpower the face, can seem to recede by using a slight bit of contour shading.

Once you've made these proportional observations, then it is a short road to looking your best.

Tinted Under Makeup Moisturizers

These special moisturizers are not necessary, but you might like to try one in place of your regular moisturizer as it can effectively alter the tone (color) of your skin. This toning is accomplished using a moisturizer which contains lightly tinted pigments and is available in liquid, cream, or gel, which are not occlusive (pore-clogging).

This type of tinted moisturizing product is used in place of or in addition to your regular moisturizer depending upon your skin type. The lollipop pastel shades of these moisturizers do not look the same as they appear in the bottle or jar once they are applied. Be sure to choose your tinted foundation very carefully to be compatible with them, so that the final effect you achieve is the desired one.

- Light sallow skin is brightened with a blue or lavender shade of moisturizer.
- A florid complexion (one that is pink, red, or looks blushed or downright ruddy) is toned down with a light green or aqua moisturizer.
- Dark sallow skin is perked up with a pink or apricot shade of moisturizer.
- Very dark or black skin having a ruddy undertone is minimized with aqua moisturizer.
- In the wide range of normal shaded complexions, a natural shade will promote a more even, allover color.

These products may be used with makeup to impart a different complexion tone than you can arrive at with just tinted foundation. They may be used without makeup as well, and in some cases this is more preferable. For example, the woman who does not wear a tinted foundation on a day-to-day basis, but needs to perk up or tone down her own skin color. If this applies to you, a moisturizer with a built-in sun screen may also be in order. No doubt, some day there will be a product of this kind that combines the two elements in one formula, and that will be individualized for different skin types for active outdoor women.

Under Eye Concealers

Almost every woman over the age of 30 has some dark circles under her eyes, and who needs them? There is a very easy, successful way to instantly be rid of them, whether you've had enough sleep or not. Using extra tinted foundation in this area will only draw attention to the circles, or cake or produce a masked effect. The only way to hide them is to use a product made for this specific purpose.

These products are a form of foundation that have a more opaque quality. They are called highlighters or concealers (the latter also known as cover-ups) and are available in cream, stick, or gel forms. The two basic names may seem to be diametrically opposed to one another, but both products serve the same purpose, at least under the eyes. However, they are not manufactured in as many shades as tinted foundations. You must select one that is two or three shades lighter than your skin tone and your foundation shade.

Apply it after your moisturizer, which makes it very easy to spread. Blend the color into the lighter surrounding areas of your skin. The effect will be a more equalized or even lighter skin tone around the eyes. By applying tinted foundation afterward, the whole effect will be one skin tone over the entire face. Now, practically speaking, you've just done away with at least five years. You may also apply a bit of the concealer to the eyelids to equalize or lighten dark lids and to act as an eye makeup base coat. Or substitute an emollient wrinkle stick for all through the day extra moisturizing or use both if one alone does not prove adequate. (There are also special products which provide the convenience of both.)

Always apply the concealer with light feather strokes, gently blending and fading out into the surrounding area. Never stretch or rub the delicate skin of the eye area when applying any type of eye makeup either under or over foundation.

A stark white highlighter used all around the eyes makes one look like a cuddly panda bear instead of a woman. Some women can wear this effectively but most cannot—it is too contrived looking. And it should never be used on puffy areas under eyes, as it will accentuate them. A natural tone of concealer is better and more natural looking under the eyes. It should be confined to the dark hollows, avoiding any puffs. (Blend *to* the puff, if you have any.) Reserve the white (preferably off-white) for just under the eyebrows and for the eyelids themselves if your eyes are small, deep-set or if you want to make your eyes appear larger.

A bit of concealer at the corners of the nose allows you to put shadows where they properly belong. Very few of us have these particular shadows in the right places and are better off putting them in ourselves. We will talk more about this under the heading of eye makeup. Naturally, if you are satisfied with the shadows at the corners of your nose, omit this step and use the concealer only under the eyes.

When attempting to cover a small, dark spot or red mark on your face, apply a tiny amount of concealer (concealing sticks closely matched to your own skin tone work best here) to the exact spot and pat it on by dabbing with one finger only. This is very important because spreading or blending will defeat your purpose. Allow to set for a few moments. Now apply your tinted foundation and very gently blend the color over those areas but make sure there is no buildup. It should be as smooth as the rest of your skin.

Some women have an unattractive dark shadow above the upper lip even though there is little or no hair in that area. A concealer in cream or stick form, closely matched to the skin tone, will effectively hide the shadow. But use sparingly and blend well, and don't use at all if there is more than just a little hair, as it will accentuate the problem.

Concealers and highlighters are somewhat opaque but are not to be confused with truly opaque products which have no transparency at all (i.e., pancake makeup) and are used to cover birthmarks, scars, and other extreme discolorations of the skin. For this purpose Lydia O'Leary's **Covermark** or Marian Bialac's **Covermark–S** very effectively disguise these areas. They are waterproof, sunproof, do not rub off, and resist cracking. If nature or fortune was unkind to you, don't be timid. A product of this type will not only make you look better, it will make you feel better. Taking care of your appearance is quite different from sheer vanity!

CONTOURING

The principle of contouring is very simple—light makes any feature come forth, dark makes it recede. You can also make undesirable features recede by highlighting other areas in order to bring them into balance. This is what we do for daytime because it is not obvious to the eye when properly blended.

Daytime

Daytime contouring requires a foundation, a highlighter, or a concealer. The foundation may be one or two shades lighter than your regular shade. It is usually a good idea to select the same brand of foundation but this is not always possible. So try to select similar consistencies if you are buying two different brands.

Just remember that the shades should be in harmony with each other. Highlighters are a little easier to select, but be sure not to get one that is too white. Stick or cream type concealers also work very well.

Concealers should be applied after moisturizer and before foundation. Highlighters and lighter foundations shades should be applied after your moisturizer and regular foundation.

Select one or two or more of these ideas, but don't go overboard. There isn't a woman alive that needs them all.

DAYTIME
USE LIGHTER SHADE ONLY

LONG OR POINTED NOSE

A single stroke down the center of nose stopping short of the tip. Leave the rounded end or point darker. Blend in.

LONG NOSE WITH CENTER BUMP

A single stroke from below the bump to tip. Blend in.

LONG NOSE WITH HIGH BRIDGE

A stroke down each side to the flare of the nose. Blend in.

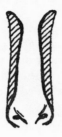

BROAD OR FLAT NOSE

A single stroke down the center of nose to the tip. Blend in.

SHORT FLAT NOSE

A generous dot, concentrating mostly on the lower bridge. Blend in.

WIDE NOSTRILS

A dot at the bridge of nose. Blend in.

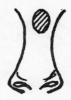

DEEP SMILE LINES FROM NOSE TO MOUTH

A single stroke on each. Blend in.

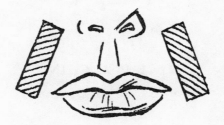

FROWN LINES BETWEEN EYEBROWS

A generous dot. Blend in.

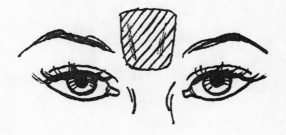

HEAVY JAWLINE

A stroke under each of your eyes blended up and over your temples. This reduces the jawline and makes it seem narrower by contrast.

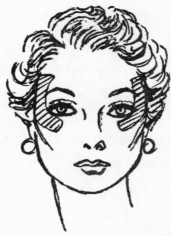

RECEDING CHIN

A generous dot over the chin and it comes forward. Blend in.

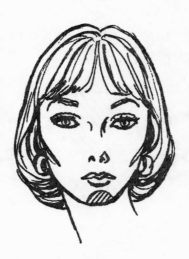

SHORT CHIN

A small dot just on the tip of chin to the indentation under the lower lip. Blend in.

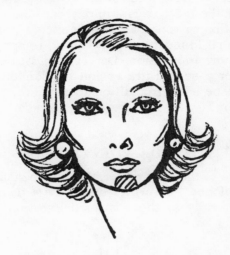

VERTICAL LINES FROM MOUTH TO NOSE

Use normal foundation or a shade lighter in this area. Blend in. Let dry, then powder. Dust away excess powder with fresh cotton, then apply lipstick.

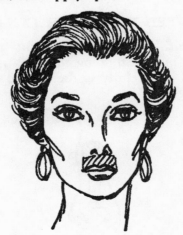

Nighttime

This kind of contouring can be very tricky in the light of day, therefore I think you ought to reserve it for evening only. The requirements are the exact reverse of daytime contouring. You will need a foundation or concealer that is one or two shades darker than your normal foundation. Concealers are applied after moisturizer and before foundation. Darker foundation shades should be applied after your moisturizer and regular foundation. These techniques can be used in addition to daytime contouring. (See pages 138–143.)

LONG OR POINTED NOSE

In addition to the light center, the darker shade is rounded on the tip of nose to further decrease its point or length. Blend in carefully so there is no delineation between the two shades.

LONG POINTED NOSE WITH CENTER BUMP

Shade bump with darker shade in addition to the lighter shade below the bump, stopping short of tip. Shade tip at the point. Blend in carefully so there is no delineation between the shadings.

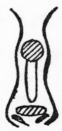

LONG NOSE WITH HIGH BRIDGE

In addition to highlighting both sides of nose, shade the bridge and tip. Blend in carefully so there are no lines of demarcation.

HUMP NOSE

Shade a narrow line down center of nose starting at where the hump begins, extending to the tip. Highlight just under the tip. Blend carefully.

ONE SIDE FULLER THAN THE OTHER

Shade the full side with contour color and use a highlighter on the narrower side. Blend both very carefully. This technique may also be used for daytime if the darker shade is very subtle.

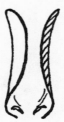

BROAD OR FLAT NOSE

In addition to the light stroke down the center, carefully blend darker shade down the sides to further reduce width.

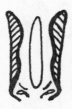

SHORT FLAT NOSE

In addition to highlighting below the bridge, shade along each side of nose to the tip of nostrils. Blend carefully.

WIDE NOSTRILS

In addition to highlighting the bridge, shade the flare on both sides of nose. Blend carefully.

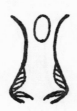

WIDE BRIDGE

The bridge will appear narrower by shading it at the sides and extending the contour color to the corners of the eyebrows. Blend carefully, removing any excess with cotton swabs. When blended carefully, this technique can also be used for daytime.

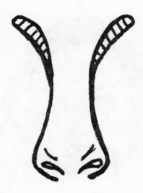

SHARP UPTURNED NOSE OR BULBOUS TIP BETWEEN NOSTRILS

Shade the tip and blend carefully.

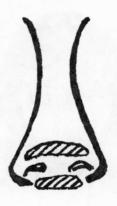

HEAVY JAWLINE

In addition to lighter shade at the temples, use a darker shade over the jawline. Be sure to blend carefully so there is no line of demarcation. You might also try this without the lighter shade to see if the effect is enough for you, but not for daytime. Daylight and indoor lighting make it too obvious unless you are really a master at it.

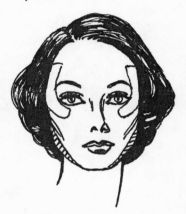

PROTRUDING CHIN

Shade under the chin and just over the tip with darker shade. Blend in.

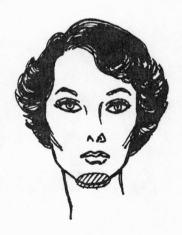

DOUBLE CHIN OR SAGGING JOWLS

Use a darker tinted foundation (a deep brownish shade of powdered blush may be substituted) under the chin and blend in slightly over the jaw. Make sure the final effect is very subtle.

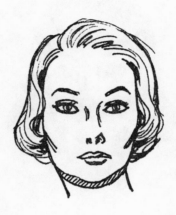

PROTRUDING UPPER LIP

Apply darker shade from the upper lip to just under the nose. Blend in.

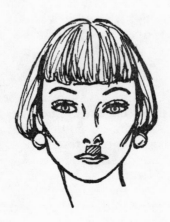

PROMINENT TEMPLES WITH HIGH FOREHEAD

Shade with darker color on the temple bones and along the hairline to de-emphasize. Blend well. A powdered blush may also be used for this purpose.

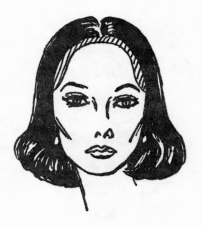

FACE SHAPES AND HAIRSTYLES

There are seven distinct facial shapes, one of which applies to every woman's face: oval; round; square; heart-shaped; diamond-shaped; long, oblong or inverted triangle; and triangular.

Oval is used as a model for it is considered the most perfect shape. All others can approximate it with a slight bit of contour shading. These techniques should only be used for nighttime when lighting is softer and more flattering. Daylight and indoor fluorescent lighting can play havoc with a cosmetically shaded face unless you are really an expert. Who knows, with enough practice you could be! But please remember, even for night, proper blending is a must so there are no lines of demarcation.

Facial contouring requires a foundation shade one or two shades darker than your regular foundation, and a highlighter. Concealing sticks will not do the job here.

Also take into consideration your hairstyle, which can give the illusion of a more perfect shape. In combination with these contouring techniques, you could have the perfect oval. If you are due for a new haircut, put yourself into the hands of a good hair stylist. The stylist will personalize your style and cut your hair, taking into consideration not only your facial shape but the special arrangement of your features, your size, your figure, whether or not you wear eyeglasses, the nature of your hair, and the life you lead. The following hairstyles in relation to facial shape are offered as a guide only.

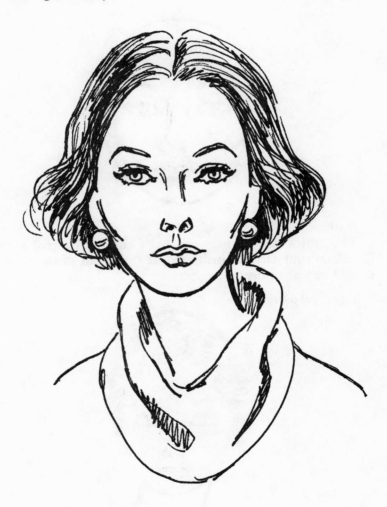

The Oval Is Your Model.

ROUND is a short, broad face with full cheeks.

Contouring:
Shade along the outer curve at the fullest part narrowing it very slightly along the chin line. Or, from the center of the cheeks to the top of the ears. Try both techniques to see which is best for you.

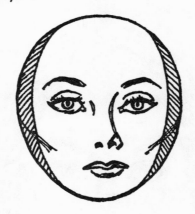

Hair:
The crown should be worn high enough to give added length to your face. In order to cut the width of the face, it should be worn close to the cheeks.

The total picture:

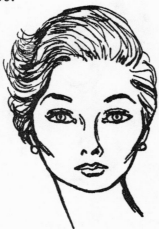

SQUARE is almost equal distance between the forehead and jawline. The sides of your face are angular.

Contouring:
Shade the corners of the jawbones and bring shading slightly upward along the outer curve.

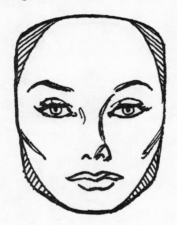

Hair:
Wear your hair softly—rounded bangs are good, so is shoulder length.

The total picture:

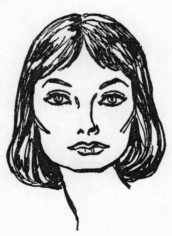

HEART-SHAPED has a wide forehead, full cheeks and/or prominent cheekbones and a narrow jaw.

Contouring:
Shade the corners of your forehead down to the top of your ears. Highlight tip of chin.

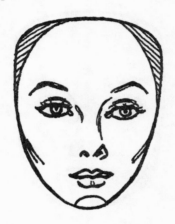

Hair:
You need to add width and fullness from the ears down. A medium length to mid-neck is good.

The total picture:

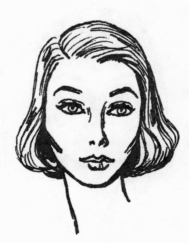

DIAMOND-SHAPED chin is pointed, and forehead and jawline are narrow. Cheekbones are wide.

Contouring:
Shade the outer curve and continue around under your chin. Highlight tip of chin and corners at the top of forehead.

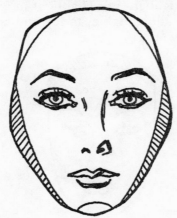

Hair:
Your hair should fall close to your cheeks. Fullness at the top with a little height will help to balance the width of your cheeks. Bangs also help to make the forehead seem broader.

The total picture:

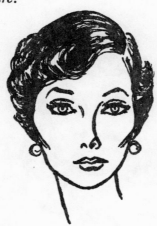

LONG, OBLONG OR INVERTED TRIANGLE face is long or thin. Forehead, cheekbones, and jawline are narrow. In the case of the inverted triangle, the forehead is wider.

Contouring:

Shade across top of forehead and tip of chin. (If tip of chin is receding then highlight it.) Highlight in front of ears or if very narrow, extend highlighter to top and bottom of shaded areas along sides of face.

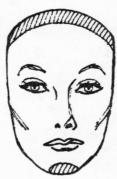

Hair:

Wear your hair full at the sides with a rounded crown. Long hair that reaches to the middle of the neck is good for you, but this isn't a hard and fast rule.

The total picture:

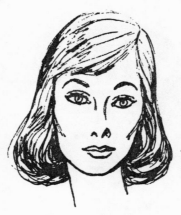

TRIANGULAR has a narrow forehead and the jawline is wider than the cheekbones.

Contouring:
Shade the fullest part of your face up to the ears. Highlight the forehead.

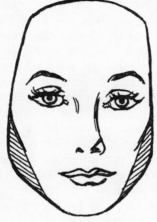

Hair:
Wear your hair wide and full at the temples, keeping it off your forehead.

The total picture:

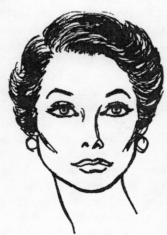

TINTED FOUNDATION
FOR A NATURAL LOOK

The most important reason for wearing a foundation is to even out your skin tone. The most beautiful skin in the world has different shades to it and benefits from this evening out.

Color and texture—in that order—are the two most important factors when buying a tinted foundation. Coverage comes third. Liquid or cream tinted foundations are the only two types that should be considered by the woman over 30, regardless of her skin type. Even oily skin benefits from a liquid foundation because it absorbs and evenly distributes excess oil. During the course of a long day, it keeps an oily skin fresher looking. At the opposite end of the spectrum, lined and crepey skin also benefits from using liquid foundation because it is less likely to form in the creases. However, these should be two different types of liquid foundation altogether. The former is a water-in-oil base and the latter is an oil-in-water base. Make sure you get the proper one for your skin type. There are other types of foundation that also have their places, but we will discuss them later.

Your tinted foundation should be extremely close to your own skin color bordering on one shade lighter. There are two reasons for this: (1) As you grow older, your own natural skin tones become a shade or two darker, and (2) indoor lighting affects the skin tone and makes it look darker.

In the course of any one day, you are outside in overcast daylight, sunlight, inside your place of business, out to lunch or to dinner, shopping, marketing, at home, and many other places, too. Your foundation shade has to look like you and your own skin under *all* these conditions. The exception is in the evenings when you want to look special and can take the time to apply a completely fresh makeup. That's when you purchase a special foundation, one that makes you look more alluring under night lights such as candlelight. This shade of foundation can be one to two shades "warmer" than your everyday foundation.

Texture should be light and sheer, taking into consideration the amount of coverage you need. And coverage depends on what you need to camouflage. Undesirable skin tones such as ruddiness, blotchy areas, pallor, or sallowness are to be considered but keep in mind, you do not want a built-up or mask-like look. Avoid

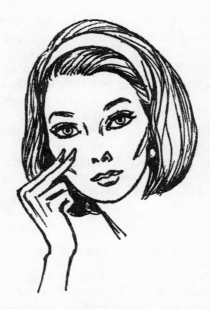

thick liquids or heavy creams. You want your base to look sheer so that your own skin is showing through. When properly applied you should be able to touch and feel true skin underneath the foundation. Foundation should not be considered a second skin. It should be a fine sheer covering for your own skin.

Applying a tinted foundation only in certain areas of the face is fine for models under the lights of the camera, where the desired result is a beautiful photograph. But, how many models are there over 30? Not many, I assure you. Unless you are one of those natural, over-30 beauties, apply your foundation all over your face, including eyelids, lips, under chin, and blend right down to the collar bone.

Apply tinted foundation with your fingertips (either middle and index or middle and ring fingers—whichever is more comfortable for you). Some women prefer a cosmetic sponge, which is fine as long as it is scrupulously cleaned, simply washed thoroughly after each use. Try both methods to discover which is best for you. (Incidentally, a silk sponge is the best.)

Blending is the spreading and thinning of any foundation. It is the all-important technique and will make the biggest difference in whether you achieve a natural or unnatural look.

You should blend so that color and consistency are evenly distributed all over your face, including eyelids—but very very thinly on the eyelids, please. Blend right into the hairline, don't worry about getting it into eyebrows or slightly into your hair because, as your next step, you are going to brush it right out. Pay particular attention to blend smoothly on nose crevices, laugh lines, around the ear lobes; smooth outward over the jawline, and go right over your lips. Continue under the chin and down the neck if you are not wearing a high neck garment.

There should be no line of demarcation where you stop—just a subtle blending, fading the edges to nothing. Use your fingertips or damp sponge, gently and evenly, no pulling, no rubbing, no undue pressure.

THE TECHNIQUES

There are two correct methods of applying foundation: The dot method is probably easiest for most women.

• Place 5 generous dots, one each on forehead, nose, cheeks, and chin. Blend these together first. When completely blended, place three more generous dots, one under the chin and two on the neck, and blend these. (Decide what you are wearing first in case you want to omit the neck, but do blend under the chin.)

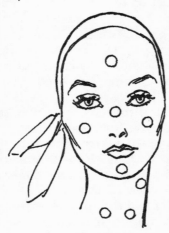

Dot Method.

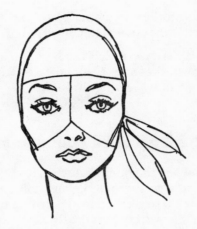

Bottle Method.

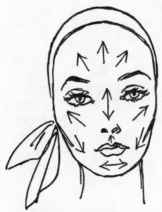

Stroke in direction of arrows.
Blend quickly but gently.

Note: A generous dot means the size of a penny. Don't be afraid to use a bit more if you feel you need it. A streaky or uneven base results from using not quite enough.

The second method is working from the bottle or jar.

• Starting at forehead, complete this area. Then apply more foundation to the nose and complete that area. On to the cheeks and eyes, blending one section into the other, then the chin and under the chin. Then the throat and neck completing each individual area before going on to the next.

It makes no difference which method you use as long as the final result is an overall evenly blended face. Remember, it should be sheer with your skin showing through.

Buying Tinted Foundations (Bases)

Foundations are the one product that women hate to buy. They complain of constantly making one color mistake after another. Let's eliminate these costly mistakes from now on.

Always use the testers practically every cosmetic company provides and never buy on the basis of how it looks in the bottle or jar. Foundations are always darker than they actually appear on your skin, and every skin wears them differently.

When you buy a foundation it would seem that the best place to test it is on your face. This is not always so because the lighting at the cosmetic counter is static and limits your viewing possibilities. Then too, you probably already have some makeup on, and this presents its own inconvenience. Certainly, it doesn't give you a true color picture when you try to put one shade over another. Then again, some women just feel awkward or undressed when applying foundation makeup in public. Yet, you need to scrutinize what you are buying closely and more important, see it under different lighting conditions. Therefore, there are several ways to go about purchasing a foundation:

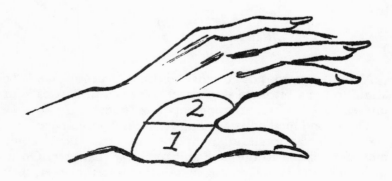

1. If you are not already wearing foundation, then try at least two of the selected shades (staying very close to your own skin tone) and apply them side by side (as in the hand illustration) to your lower cheek area. Blend each shade to a sheer consistency. Look at them in the mirror under the lights at the cosmetic counter. You are most likely looking at them under soft incandescent lighting (which is more flattering than other lighting). Now, walk away—you can very nicely explain to the lady behind the counter that you want to observe the shades under other lights and will return shortly. Go to another area of the store where the lighting is different. You will probably find fluorescent lighting in the very next department. Look at the shades on your face in several different mirrors. Since cosmetic counters are usually on the main floor or at street level, convenient to daylight, just walk outside and observe the shades in daylight (make sure you have a good size mirror with you). Observing in daylight is the most important of all. It is the true, final, test—what looks good in natural daylight looks good anywhere!

2. If you are wearing foundation but don't have any on your neck (which is even a better test site for the woman who refuses to continue her foundation down on her neck regardless of her neckline clothing), use the neck area for testing two selected foundation shades that will best match the skin color of your neck. Blend them to a sheer consistency and then follow the above walking procedure.

3. If you feel that the above method is disturbing to your appearance (even though you ordinarily wear foundation on your neck), or just don't like the inconvenience it presents, then apply a dab of each foundation shade to the back of your hand between your thumb and index finger as illustrated. The color and texture here are closest to that of your face. Blend to a sheer consistency. Follow the above walking procedure. With this procedure, you have an extra advantage because you have more opportunity to observe.

4. If the back of your hand is mottled at the test site, or if you feel for some reason it does not offer a good test, then use the inside of your wrist. Blend both shades to a sheer consistency and follow the above walking procedure.

The longer you have your two test shades on, the more they

have a chance to dry. This gives you the opportunity to see the true color and how it will eventually look on your face, especially in natural daylight. Then make your selection. Stay away from anything that looks muddy on your skin. Buy it only if you are convinced that it looks like your skin tone—but better!

That takes care of color and for the most part, consistency. But what about consistency? You should be able to use and apply your tinted foundation directly to your face without the bother and time-consuming effort of having to dilute or alter it in any way. There are enough brands on the market to choose from for the right consistency and coverage for you. Every formulation is somewhat different from company to company (with various formulas within a company). Let's face it, cosmetic chemists have the expertise and the laboratory conditions to control the minute subtleties in a formula that we couldn't possibly hope to attain by mixing our own, especially on a day in, day out basis. However, in some rare instances when one has hit on what seems to be the perfect shade but the consistency is just a bit too heavy, lending slightly more coverage than is needed for a sheer, "true skin" look, put the tiniest drop of moisturizer (if your skin leans towards the dry) or the merest drop of skin freshener (if your skin leans toward the oily) into the palm of your hand and mix it with your foundation and then apply it to your face. This takes a little longer to blend properly on the face and it is important to remember that the final result must be an overall, evenly blended complexion. My advice is to seek out the brand that gives you all three—color, texture (consistency), coverage—remember, in that order. If you shop wisely, your skin will truly look beautiful.

TINTED FOUNDATION (BASE): SHADE GUIDE

The following shade guide is by no means a final answer. There are just too many shades which you must try. It is offered only as a guide.

Fair Skin   contains hues of blue, a slightly yellow tinge, slightly pink, or just plain white. Foundation should be in the category of light beige, bisque or ivory or one with a pink tint.

Ruddy Skin	contains pink, red, rose, or brownish-red hues. Foundation should be in the category of beige to tan with only a slight rose tint. (If very ruddy, eliminate rose tint.)
Sallow Skin	contains yellow, green, or grey hues. Foundation should be in the category of rose or peach. For a golden look, amber or honey shades.

If skin is very pale and hair is graying or white, choose a foundation shade one shade darker than your own skin tone. One with a pink cast will be very pretty on you.

There are at least 35 different hues to black skin, and therefore, black women must be extremely selective when purchasing a tinted foundation. Sometimes, a mixture of two foundation shades will produce the shade that will be right for your skin, if you cannot find one that is to your liking. But do stay close to your own skin tone or try to match the foundation shade to your skin's underlying tones whether it is blue, yellow, or orange. Use the "walking" procedure outlined on page 162 before you buy to avoid making a double expense mistake.

Take into consideration the seasons of the year. If you like to have fun in the sun, you'll need a different tint to enhance your skin. Fall clothing after a summer's normal exposure—just being outdoors—requires a reappraisal of your foundation shade, even if you don't tan. Hopefully, you wear a good sunblock and don't deliberately sunbathe (see page 26). Spring brings with it pastel colors in the clothes you wear, and a slight adjustment of the tint may be in order. But remember, always stay as close to your own skin tone as possible. Remember too, that for everyday-wear some brands of foundation (moisturizers also) contain sun-screens. These are great for the woman who has sensitive-to-sunlight or delicate skin. Or, for the woman who just wants to preserve her skin if she spends more than a little time outdoors.

Types of Tinted Foundations

The all-in-one foundation available in a dry compact form is actually both liquid and powder compressed into a cake, and usually packaged in a pretty compact. It is used as quick makeup when time does not permit the use of your regular foundation, such as in a quick getaway in the morning. Or, it is used as a touch-up when time does not permit a complete re-do if your makeup is past touching up with a translucent powder.

Compressed translucent powders are packaged similarly, but they are powders without tint or a base of their own. They take the place of loose powder but are more convenient to carry with you for they are also packaged in a compact. They are used to touch up a complete makeup during the course of the day, to remove shine from nose, chin, or under eyes, or for powdering lips in preparation for lipstick after one has eaten.

Solid cream foundations are opaque and are only recommended for blemishes that appear under the skin or broken veins. Cream-sticks or pancake foundations can give a pasty or heavy appearance. They are sometimes successfully used when one has deep-pitted scars left over from the teenage acne years. They are used with a damp sponge, but a combination of your fingertips and a sponge achieves the most satisfactory blend for the creamstick type foundation. A rather moist sponge works best with the pancake type. Work a small area with only a small amount of pancake on the sponge at any time. When completed, go over the entire face and neck gently with the damp sponge to even out the makeup and remove any excess.

Tube types that are a mixture of semi-liquid and powder usually have a matte (non-shiny) finish. They are applied with fingertips or sponge. They are recommended only for oily skin, but a water-in-oil liquid is still superior and should be your first choice. The tube types are more difficult to apply because they require fast blending. Medicated foundations are for blemished skin. They conceal while they help to heal, but they should definitely not be worn in the sun (see page 29).

Special Notes on Foundation and Powder

Lipstick "bleeding" into fine lines around the mouth can virtually be prevented by applying liquid foundation, allowing it to dry, and lightly fluffing powder over this area before applying lipstick.

Fine lines around your eyes will appear to be reduced by applying liquid foundation, allowing it to dry, and then fluffing on powder. Using a clean cotton ball or a special fine-bristle powder brush, whisk away any excess powder. A matte finish in these areas makes them look far less conspicuous. Besides, powder helps to hold any eye makeup that would ordinarily smudge onto other areas of the face. This is quite prevalent in some women.

Facial hair or down on the lower portion of the face is also less conspicuous when you use very gentle downward strokes to flatten the hair. (This is one of those rare exceptions when you use downward strokes and it should be confined to that area and purpose only.)

If you're trying to conceal freckles, use a second application of your foundation in freckled areas only, after the first has completely dried.

Trying to conceal a flat mole? Use a stick type concealer on that area only. It may take two applications. Remove any excess in surrounding area with cotton swab. Then apply your foundation. Trying to conceal a raised mole? See your dermatologist for possible removal.

Foundation will not rub off onto your clothing from your neck if you powder and blot with tissue, or damp sponge it when the entire makeup is completed.

Remember to shake the bottle! Even though many liquid foundations are homogenized, it is always best to be sure the mixture has not separated. After applying your foundation, clean out corners of eyes and the tips of nostrils with cotton swabs.

Apply crayon type of eyebrow pencil after your foundation. The foundation allows you to correct any excess with a cotton swab because you have the proper amount of "slip," just in case one eyebrow gets thicker than the other.

If you do not wear powder (I hope to convince you differently before you finish this book) then blot nose and chin with tissue after foundation is completely dry.

And most important of all, let your foundation *dry* before proceeding with powder or eye makeup. A full explanation of this will be given with the discussion of face powders (page 181).

BLUSHER OR ROUGE

There is one subject about which I definitely agree with the models and actresses who claim that a blusher is the one cosmetic they most rely on. I too, believe it is the one makeup item that is truly indispensable for all women. If I were at sea and had to abandon ship for the lifeboat and could only grab one color cosmetic on the way (notice, I said "color"), it would have to be my blusher. If I could only take one "item" with me it would be my moisturizer. Naturally, I'm assuming I have my lifejacket first!

A blush of color on the cheeks can do more for any woman than any other color cosmetic, including lipstick. It perks up, lifts up, and brightens any complexion, makes one look healthy, defines good cheekbones, brings out cheekbones where they didn't seem to exist, even brightens the eyes by contrast. But like any other cosmetic it can be overused, its purpose misunderstood, it can even create a clown appearance.

A blusher should be used for the purpose it was intended, to heighten and brighten the cheeks with color. Lately it seems to have been pirated for other areas of the face. It has certain advantages but they should be used sparingly and kept to a minimum by the woman over 30. The eye travels toward rouged areas of the face, so it can easily point up flaws or features you would rather hide.

A common mistake women make with blush or rouge is to blend it too close to the eye area, even getting it into the fine lines there, which accentuates their existence. Blending it too close to the nose will make any finely shaped nose look distorted, so you can imagine what it does to a nose that is not quite so finely shaped! And blush or rouge should never appear below the level of the nostrils. Keeping these few no-nos in mind, it is really very easy to place rouge on the cheeks to result in a natural looking glow.

Look into your mirror and smile very broadly, making a forced grin. Really smile tightly, which puffs out your cheeks. At the point of the most rounded flesh—you might call it the high point or the apple of the cheek—place a dot or two of color on the center, dead center. Hold the forced grin for a few seconds so that when you start blending the color doesn't creep into the smile lines between nose and mouth or travel down too low on the cheek. Blend upward and outward towards the ears but no higher than where the top of the ear is connected to the face and no lower than the earlobes. Blend almost to your hairline, fading the edges into the hairline to make it look like a natural glow ema-

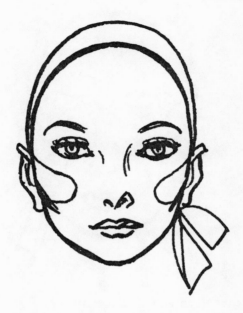

nating from the head. Repeat on the other cheek. The darkest portion of color should either be near the hairline or at the center of the cheekbones, but it should not look like a blob of color, just a subtle blending. This same technique works for any face type because you are placing it on your natural bone structure, which is where smiling Mother Nature would place it and this automatically creates hollows where they naturally exist.

Hollowing the cheekbones for a heightened dramatic effect is something else. For that effect, you place a darker or brownish shade of blusher (sometimes referred to as contour color, which can be a cream or a powder) in the hollows of the cheeks, confining the color to that area alone. The easiest way to do this is to suck in your cheeks. Use only the smallest dot of color and carefully blend one color into the other so that there is no line of demarcation between the two shades of rouge. (Between applica-

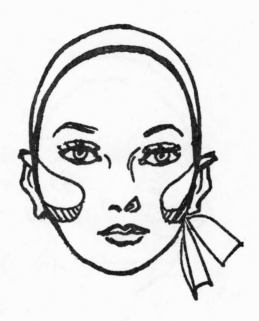

tions, make sure to wipe your fingertips of excess color on a damp sponge or hand towel. This holds true whenever changing from one color to another anywhere on the face.) Blend the darker, hollowing shade outward to the ear but not lower than the earlobe. The exceptions are a square or triangular shaped face in which cases color may be brought down lower than the earlobes.

Remember, one procedure is for health, the other is for hollows, and if you want to, you can have both at the same time.

OTHER USES FOR BLUSHER OR ROUGE

• A slight touch at the hairline in the case of a too high forehead helps to diminish its prominence. If you are tired or depressed a mere touch of color at the temples gives an extra lift.

• A slight bit of brownish blush on tip of nose or edge of chin will shorten its appearance.

• Applying blush on earlobes adds width to the face, but it also calls attention to the earlobes in case yours are not too pretty and you would rather they were less conspicuous.

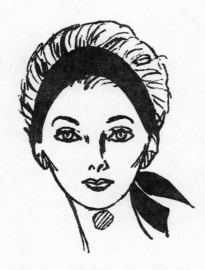

• A mere touch on the center of the neck, well blended, helps to make the head and neck look like they belong to each other.

In using any of the above techniques, remember to apply the blush sparingly and blend well.

Every woman who uses cream, liquid, or gel blushers should also own a powdered blusher to add an extra dash of color when her entire makeup is completed. This is a sometime thing, but the occasion does arise, especially when a garment is chosen or changed at the last minute. Liquid, cream, or gel blushers should not be used as a finishing touch as they will not do justice to your newly completed makeup when just that extra small touch of color is needed.

Also, please remember that cream, gel, or liquid blushers are applied after foundation to protect your skin. (The foundation acts as a buffer.) Dry or powdered blushes are applied over foundation *and* powder if face powder is used on the cheek area, or over foundation alone if it is the only type blush used. Glosses are applied over foundation using no powder in that area.

SHADE GUIDE

Fair complexions	Pink, coral, or tawny tones
Medium complexions	Peach, rose, tawny, or red tones
Medium to dark complexions	Tawny or deep wine tones
Dark or sallow complexions	Clear red tones
Ruddy complexions	Peach, deep wine, or russet tones
Suntanned complexions	Bright corals, deep copper tones
Black complexions	Clear red, bronze or russet tones
All complexions under night lights (with the exception of ruddy)	Rose or warm red tones

TYPES OF BLUSHER OR ROUGE

CONSISTENCY	APPLICATION AND RELATIVE AMOUNT
Creams are packaged in small jars, pans, compacts, sticks, tubes, or crayons. They are probably the easiest to use for most women.	Apply a small dot or two.
Gels are packaged in squeeze tubes.	Apply a tiny dot or two.
Liquids are packaged in small bottles. Some have a self-measuring device which can be handy as liquid rouge has a tendency to spread and dry very fast.	Apply a teeny dot or two.
Glosses are usually packaged in large swivel sticks and contain little or no color of their own. They are finishing touches. If you want to make the apple of the cheek to appear larger, a gloss finisher is your desired product.	Apply in one or two strokes.

Dry, cake, or solid (all the same type) are usually supplied with a small puff.

Make sure puff is not overloaded with color. Apply in light sweeping motions.

Powdered or cake supplied with brush are usually matte finishes and are best if you want to make the apple of the cheek appear smaller. There are also frosted shades in this type product which are better for evening wear.

Make sure brush is not overloaded and apply with light sweeping motions.

EYEBROWS REFLECT OUR CHARACTER!

Eyebrows have the ability to express our thoughts more than any other of our features. The eyes may be windows of the soul

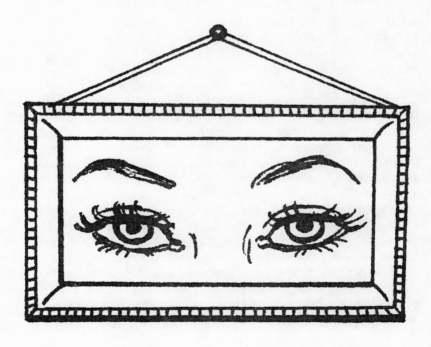

but the eyebrows reflect our emotions more quickly and accurately. Just think of how your brows go up when you are surprised!

The eyebrows should be frames for the eyes. They should not be contoured to conform to the shape of the face although this naturally comes into play when brows are properly framed for the eyes. They should not be overwhelmingly thick so that they close in the eyes, nor should they be so thin that you are constantly registering a look of amazement. The eyebrows should not detract from the eyes, they should simply compliment them. (See pages 105–107 for eyebrow shaping.)

Most of us need some penciling-in on the eyebrows to compensate for what may be lacking or to correct the contour. If you are one of those lucky ladies who have natural brows that only require a little tweezing to maintain their shape, don't indulge in the use of eyebrow makeup. Just brush them into place. The rest of us will have to emulate your good fortune by penciling-in the few tiny hair strokes that seem to be missing.

And that's what penciling-in is: a few tiny hair strokes to resemble natural hairs. They are drawn with the point of a very sharp eyebrow pencil, following the natural or the corrected-to-appear-natural eyebrow contours, which in turn, follow the bone structure of the eyes. If anything makes a woman look harsh and unappealing, it is the heavy penciled-in line that appears to frame her face instead of her eyes in a most unflattering way.

The easiest way to apply these tiny strokes with an eyebrow pencil is right after you have completed the blending of your foundation and rouge. It is at this point that you have the right amount of slip to draw these tiny lines. Just in case of error, they can be easily erased with a cotton swab without upsetting your foundation or any other makeup you may have previously applied. In addition your eyebrows are already properly placed to provide guidelines for the application of eye shadow that follows. It is now advantageous to brush the tinted foundation (which provided extra control of unruly hairs) out of the brows. If your foundation provides too much slip, then wait until it has dried before applying your eyebrow pencil. If this still proves to be too much slip, then apply your eyebrow pencil after your face powder, then lightly dust the eyebrows with powder to remove excess shine of the crayon. This is advantageous even if you do not normally wear face powder.

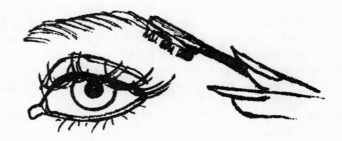

Before applying eyebrow pencil, brush the hairs downward with your eyebrow brush. This will facilitate your drawing of the tiny hairlike strokes. Start no further in than the inside corner of the eye, curving the hairlike strokes to the peak (which should be in line with the outside of the iris) and terminating no further than the outside corner of the eye. You can easily check this with the folded paper method described on pages 105–106. It might be a good idea to leave the folded paper on your dressing table as part of your equipment. It will help make your efforts consistent from day to day. I know many women whose eyebrows never seem to look the same way twice due to their inability to halt the line at the proper place.

Always end the brow line with a slightly upward tilt. This little lift is very important to the character of the face. But go carefully, too much of an upward tilt is unnatural, an occurrence with many women who tend to overdo.

Now brush the eyebrow hairs upward lightly to control the line. A light dusting of powder over the brows will set them for the

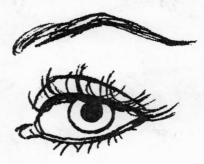

day. Should you get a little too much powder on, give them an additional light brushing. Again, be sure not to use a heavy hand as this will blur the hairline strokes into a continuous line—the big no-no! The use of powder not only sets the pencilled-in brows but they won't be so quick to rub off in the dentist's chair or other daily activities. The powder also helps to tone down the somewhat greasy sheen that all eyebrow pencils leave which really looks unnatural.

Powdered eyebrow makeup takes the place of an eyebrow pencil. This is available in cake form and is supplied with a brush whose tip is angled to facilitate the same drawing-in of tiny stroked lines. It is best applied after powdering as its components tend to be somewhat fly-away, but do not require an additional powdering since it is a powder to begin with. Otherwise, use powdered eyebrow makeup in the same manner as you would an eyebrow pencil. The effect is somewhat different, the pencil being more definite, the powder being softer.

Colors should be soft and chosen to compliment your hair. Avoid black unless you are a really dramatic brunette type, and even then it should only be softly applied. Colors do not have to be the exact shade of your hair, but should be in harmony with its color and at least one shade lighter than the hairs of your eyebrows. A darker shade than your hair produces an aged appearance.

Remember too, that pencil color shows up darker when applied. To compensate for this, you may find that using two different colored pencils will give you a more natural effect. For example, a woman with medium brown hair and eyebrows might use light brown and medium brown pencils. Of course, this is op-

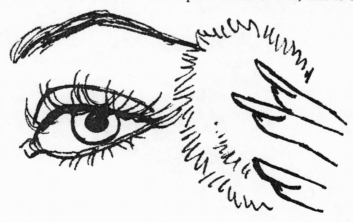

tional, but for some women it works very well, especially when one doesn't seem to hit upon that one right shade. Redheads often have this problem.

If you wear eyeglasses, don't try to compensate your eyebrows for the glasses you wear. Keep the brow line where it naturally belongs. Trying to extend it over the rim to make yourself appear to have brows, creates an unnatural look. Have no doubts. They are seen when your face is at a ¾ angle or in profile.

Keep your eyebrow pencil sharp. If it does not have a built-in sharpener, buy a small separate one made for this express purpose. It is much easier, quicker, and safer to use than a razor blade.

SHADE GUIDE

HAIR COLOR	RANGE OF PENCIL OR POWDER COLORS (pencil may also be used with powder when mixing—use both sparingly)
Light blondes	Ash blonde (gold for evening only)
Medium blondes	Ash blonde, light brown (or a mix of both and/or gold for evening)
Dark blondes	Light brown (may be mixed with grey, lightly)
Light brownettes	Light brown (may be mixed with medium grey)
Medium brownettes	Light brown, medium brown (or a mix of both)
Dark brunettes	Medium brown, dark brown, charcoal (or a mix of two)
Jet black	Charcoal grey, dark brown, black (or a mix of two and silver for evening)
Light redheads	Ash blonde, auburn (or a mix of both and/or gold for evening)
Medium redheads	Auburn, light brown (or a mix of both)
Dark redheads	Auburn, light brown, medium brown (or a mix of auburn and medium brown)
Grey or silver	Grey, charcoal grey (may be mixed with light brown or silver for evening)

FACE POWDER:
THE LEAST UNDERSTOOD COSMETIC

Powder has virtues that are greatly underestimated. Lots of women say, "I like a dewy look," but many do not really understand what a dewy look is. They think the use of powder will totally obscure the glow and freshness of what they hope appears more youthful. This is especially true in women over 40.

Let's see what a dewy look really is and what it is not. A dewy look is a radiant glow where some areas of the face appear moist and other areas appear matte. Dew on the petal of a flower is never all over the petal—that's just wetness. Dew is sprinkled in droplets on the petals, and the flower appears to have both wet and dry areas. Could it be that this is one of the reasons everyone thinks flowers are beautiful? A dewy look is *not* a shiny, wet, oily, or greasy look all over the face. Yet there are many women who display this appearance.

There are natural areas of the face that should appear moist, namely the cheeks and sides of the forehead. On *some* women the tip of the chin looks pretty when it appears slightly moist. The various lighting we are all seen under plays a tremendous part in this. A complexion which has an allover shine is competing with the shine of the eyes, the shine of the lipstick, and the shine of the cheeks. Too much for any one face, don't you think?

Powder reflects light! You know, the one thing we never really see with our own eyes is our own face. Think about it for a mo-

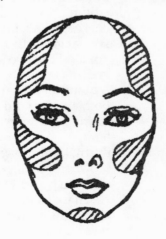

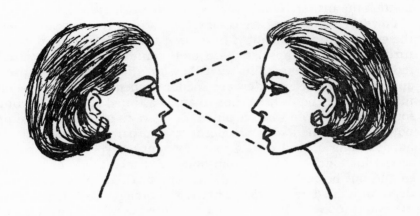

ment. We can easily look at our own hands, legs, feet, any part of our anatomy, except our faces. If it were not for mirrors we would never even know what we look like. Naturally, we can't carry a mirror in front of us all the time to see how we look under the lights that play upon our faces and the shadows they create. If we could, we would see a multitude of distortions. Even a perfect nose can look ill-proportioned when certain lights are cast on it. Average-sized pores can appear enlarged. Tiny, tiny lines under the eyes can look like cracks in the skin. The under-eye area is a most unnatural place for shine—it detracts from the shine of the eyes, besides appearing age inducing. Allow me to qualify this viewpoint as it is certain to meet with some opposition. I remain steadfast in the conviction that shine under the eyes is age inducing but you may very likely question the use of face powder in this area. It is really a matter of technique! If you dust translucent powder on very lightly and whisk away any excess with clean cotton or dab with damp sponge it should not cake or form in those tiny lines or creases. If it does, then by all means omit it, but do not compensate by using a foundation that has less sheen and more matte finish. But please retain this perspective—an all-powdered or all-matte look over the entire face can make it look flat and uninteresting.

The whole principle of makeup is counterpoint: light and shadow; sheen and matte; play up the good features and play down the bad; accentuate the positive and if we can't eliminate, at least minimize the flaws. Obviously, a combination of moist and matte is the answer. That's what powder is all about!

Powders themselves have come a long way in recent years. Even the good old tinted standbys have been further refined and moisturized (micro-encapsulated). Don't confuse this with actual moisturizing for your skin—what they do is impart a moisturized appearance. Tinted powders are fine for women who still refuse or insist that they don't have time to apply a tinted foundation. But for the woman who wears a tinted foundation, her only choice in powder should be loose translucent or transparent powder, which have no color of their own. Pressed or compact types should be reserved for touch-ups away from home. A tinted shade of powder should not be added to tinted foundation. Color plus color produces unwanted results, particularly the orangey look that everyone wants to avoid. If you *must* wear tinted powder, at least make sure it exactly matches the tone of your foundation but is one or two shades lighter. There are also translucent powders that provide only luminosity (glow finish) and can be used by themselves or in combination with a matte translucent powder. (Example: A luminescent powder may be used on the cheek area and sides of forehead and a translucent/transparent powder on the rest of the face.)

There are still more virtues of powder that you should know about. Powder sets and holds your entire makeup for the day. It gives it a finished, flawless look by refining the skin's texture. A mere touch-up hours later will make you look almost as fresh as when you first applied it. Powdering the lips provides a base and holds lipstick on longer; it also keeps it from bleeding into fine lines around the lips. Powdering the eyelids and eyelashes provides a base for eyeshadow and mascara, and the lashes appear thicker and longer (even more so, if you apply a bit of petroleum jelly to the lashes before powdering). Powder also helps to hold the mascara for hours longer. Last, but not least, it minimizes the sheen of greasy eyebrow pencils.

MOIST + MATTE = DEWY

There are several techniques used to achieve the moist and matte look and I hope you'll choose one of them. They have various degrees of matte so if you are one who still clings to the no-powder look, there is a special method for you to achieve the bare minimum with the most sheen.

There is one important point that is part of my technique which should be emphasized at this time. The finished surface is what is important for appearance, as well as for how long your makeup will last. This is one of the most common mistakes because it is one of the least known techniques in makeup. It is very important to allow a lapse of time between the final blending of foundation (including blush or rouge) and the application of face powder. This interlude is what really sets your makeup to last and to appear fresh and clean for the entire day.

Don't worry, you are not going to sit there idle during this lapse. The time is utilized to brush eyebrows into place and to apply eyebrow pencil if needed, and most of us do. Note that if you use eyebrow powder (cake) you should apply after face powder. (See page 176.) Now is a good time to arrange your hair and carefully brush the hairline to whisk away any excess makeup. By the time you have combed and brushed your hair, your makeup will be dry and powder should then be applied—not a minute sooner. If your hair is very short or is easy to arrange, use the time to put on your pantyhose, bra, make the bed, read the morning

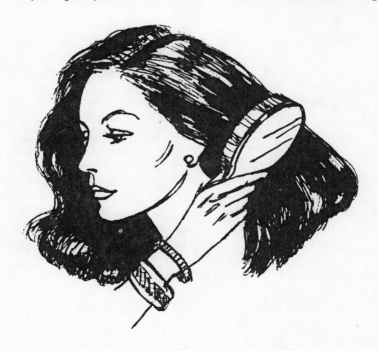

mail, whatever! Just make sure that the foundation is no longer tacky to the touch. (Important note: if you use rouge of any type other than dry or powdered blush, it should go on directly after you have finished blending your foundation and the two should be regarded as one. They will dry and set together.)

Tinted face powder should not be used over tinted foundation. It is best used over moisturizer or over foundation having no color of its own. This is not considered a complete makeup but is useful sometimes when one is in a hurry. Make sure to dust away any excess with a fresh piece of cotton or special sable powder brush.

TRANSLUCENT OR TRANSPARENT POWDERS

To *press* powder is to dab with light but firm motions. To *dust* powder is to fluff it on with light sweeping motions. (See pages 8–9 if further clarification is needed.) The two methods result in two different appearances, the latter having more sheen. But powder will last longer with the press method.

Luminescent (glow finishing) powders may be substituted. Frosted (pearl, silver, or gold flecked) powders are for evening wear.

Technique 1	Press powder over entire face and under chin and neck, omitting cheek area and sides of forehead. Dust lightly over eyelids and under eyes.
Technique 2	Press powder over entire face, under chin and neck, but omit cheek area and sides of forehead. Then dust lightly over cheeks, forehead, eyelids, and under eyes. Or substitute luminescent or frosted powder and dust the cheeks and sides of forehead to highlight them.
Technique 3	Press in the T-zone only from the center of the forehead down to nose, mouth, and chin. Dust under eyes. Pressing powder in under chin and neck is optional.
Technique 4	Press powder on nose and mouth. Eyes and under chin and neck are optional.
Technique 5	Press or dust powder on nose only.

Too many choices? Try one a day for the next week and then decide which is best for you.

For the dust technique, a long handled powder brush with full, fluffy, long bristles is fine if it is kept in immaculate condition. Admittedly a brush of this type is more difficult to maintain because of the buildup of powder over a period of time. I think it is better to reserve its use for whisking away excess powder. These brushes (especially sable, which is still the best) are quite costly and repeated cleanings will ruin fine bristles. When you do find it necessary to clean, dip it in 70 percent alcohol and wipe with tissue, then set aside to dry in open air.

For application of both dust and press techniques, a powder puff achieves the best results and should be your first preference. You should always use a clean puff, but clean cotton is preferable to a dirty powder puff.

A dirty velour powder puff is hand washable. Let it dry without squeezing the water out. This picks up the nap and makes it rough. It may take two days or more to dry but it is worth it—otherwise you would probably have to discard it. A minute or two in the dryer will fluff it up almost as good as new.

The final touch is optional. Using a silk, natural or cosmetic sponge or a cotton pad or ball, wring it out in cool water and very lightly dab all over the face and neck. Make sure that most of the water is squeezed out.

By now you have probably noticed that cotton is a prime material for both cleansing and making up. I would like to offer a suggestion: When you have your necessary tools readily accessible, it makes life so much easier, if you stuff a good size quantity of cotton or cotton balls into a large jar and keep it on your dressing table or wherever you make up, you'll then find it a breeze to move quickly through your routine. An apothecary jar is not only pretty, but ideal for this purpose regardless of the form in which you buy your cotton—balls, pads, or rolls. (In the latter case, spend a minute and tear off individual wads, refilling as necessary from the package.) I've examined the dressing rooms of many a lady, and when she has to dig into a drawer to get out that large bag of cotton balls or to pull out that big roll from a cabinet, she'll just as soon skip it—only because it is so annoying and such a waste of time. Make it easy for yourself!

Eye Makeup:
Every Woman Is
an Artist

This is where my personal expertise shines most—it should! I introduced and marketed much of the eye makeup of the late 1950s, which introduced *en masse* for the average American woman the concept of wearing colored eyeshadow and eyeliner on an everyday basis. At that time, women who used more than just a bit of mascara and eyebrow pencil were considered theatrical types. I am probably best remembered in the cosmetic industry for innovation. I invented the concept and was first to market the liquid eyeliner nationally. These then new products started the ball rolling and burgeoned into the fantastic industry eye makeup comprises today—a business within a business. The use of these products has never gone out of style since the late 50s, but it certainly did change in concept many times over. When I first introduced the liquid eyeliner, it was intended to be a fine line drawn at the base of the eyelids to make the eyes look larger and the lashes appear longer, thicker, and to delicately reshape the contours of the eyelids to more perfect proportions. But whatever happened to it during the 1960s? Remember the heavy Cleopatra eyes, the elongated upturned wings? It went through various other style changes too, and happily we have come full circle back again to the natural look. But did you know that makeup, and particularly eye makeup, is an enchanting part of history? Man, in the true

sense of the word, has been painting his body since time imme-
morial. Since earliest recorded history, both sexes have sought to
make themselves look neat, well groomed, and attractive to the
eye. The word cosmetic comes from the ancient Greek word *Kos-
mos,* meaning adornment.

The Greeks were more or less indifferent to makeup, they had
loftier aspirations. But they admired the Etruscan woman who had
equal status with men. The Etruscans left demonstrable proof of
their interest in cosmetics in the form of mirrors, utensils for the
nails, beautiful cosmetic boxes and flasks, and spatulas which they
used to apply rouge.

The Romans assimilated their ideas on makeup from Egypt, but
it was the Cretans (whose island in the northern Mediterranean
bridged both Greek and Roman cultures with Egypt) who were
the forerunners of cosmetics in the sense we know them today.
From that time to the 20th century there was not significant ad-
vancement in cosmetics' form.

It was the royal ladies of the palace of Crete (circa 1600 B.C.)
who used black incense (kohl) to underline their eyes. Frankly, it
was this knowledge coupled with watching my sister struggling to
apply eyebrow pencil to her huge eyes (she wanted to reduce the
size of her eyelids) , that gave me the idea to create an easy flowing
liquid eyeliner for the upper eyelids to minimize or maximize
their size and shape. My thought at the time was that *under*lining
the eyes in severe, dark, thick lines, all the way to the inner corners
closed the eyes in—and I still think so! The company I worked for
at the time was Lilly Daché Cosmetics (she was the famous hat
designer whose company later went into cosmetics) . And, it was
the executive head of the company, Rolf Warner, who gave me

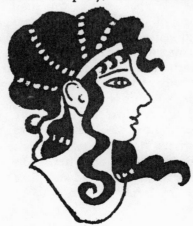

free license to work with the laboratory to develop this product. I
am still eternally grateful to him. Subsequently, I went back to
Revlon and was responsible for marketing their eyeliners (which
now also included pencils specifically formulated for the eyelids)
and the first completely coordinated line of eye makeup, which
swept a major portion of the female population of this country
and the world into a new cosmetic habit. Helena Rubinstein had
just marketed the first automatic mascara wand, called Mascara-
matic. There was always intense rivalry between Revlon and
Rubinstein (also a constant interchange of executive personnel)
as to who would market a product first. In this case, Revlon lost,
but we immediately followed with a slightly different version
called Roll-On Mascara, which eventually became generic. I as
well as others could readily forecast the coming revolution, for the
whole industry was to jump on the bandwagon. While it has become a part of makeup history, it is the 20th century that is really
more interesting. Particularly the late 1970s when every woman's
eyes can be alluring, tantalizing, and natural all at the same time.

INDIVIDUALIZED EYE MAKEUP
FOR 25 EYE SHAPES

First decide which of the following eye shapes best describes the
shape or special problem feature of your eyes—there are 25 different ones. We will then discuss each product individually, but there
is one beauty rule that applies to almost every woman's eyes. That
is, do not close the eyes in by underlining the lower eyelids in
dark brown or black. There are a few exceptions, but they apply
only to certain eye shapes, and as you shall see, these shapes are
indicated. Instead of dark brown or black, you will find blue
softer and it really makes the whites of the eyes look whiter regardless of the color of your eyes. Use a deep shade of blue, one
with a grayish cast. Also, try starting at the outside corner of the
eye and work inward. I know you're probably used to starting at
the inside corner, but this is a prettier effect and once you try it,
I think you will agree. With this technique you are less likely to
draw a thick heavy line, also less likely to bring it all the way
to the inside corners (more about that later). You can stop the
line on the lower lids almost anywhere along the way but for certain shapes I have made suggested stopping points to acquire the
maximum aesthetic effect.

CREATING LARGER EYES

Use offwhite eyeshadow over the eyelids and a light taupe blended from the crease out to the brows. Use deep brown in the crease of the lids. Shade a bit of brown at the inside corners. Remove excess with cotton swab and soften the line. Use eyeliner in a thin ribbon across the entire lids. Underline the eyes in blue. Mascara all of the upper and lower lashes.

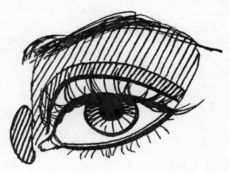

TO ENHANCE NORMAL EYES AND MAKE THEM APPEAR ALMOND SHAPED

Use a light beige or taupe (or any other light shade) eyeshadow over the entire lid. Use deep brown in the creases. Use liner and mascara only on the outer half of both upper and lower lids giving a slight lift to the corners (not up-turned wings). Underline the outer half of lower lids with blue.

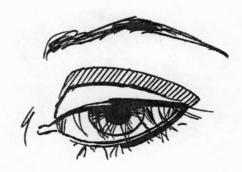

TO PLAY UP SMALL EYES

Use light shades of eyeshadow from the base of the lashes to the crease, and then up and out with darker smoky shades. Line the upper lids very thinly and close to the base of the lashes (see pages 203–204 for technique). Underline barely from outer corners to center of pupils. A touch of white at the outer corners further enlarges them. Use mascara on upper lashes only.

TO BRING OUT DEEP-SET EYES

Use a light shade of eyeshadow over the entire eyelids including inside corners. Blend it into a deep curve to the crease. Use a darker eyeshadow above the crease to the brows gradually fading out the color as it nears them. Blend outward to corners. Use a still darker shadow in the crease. (This is optional but it further brings out the eyes.) Use eyeliner only at the center of the lids and omit underlining. Use mascara lightly, concentrating mostly on the tips of lashes.

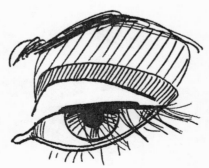

TO BRING OUT SHALLOW EYES

Use a deep tone eyeshadow such as dark taupe or brown, apply over the lids at the center, and blend out to just below the brows. Use any pale shade over the rest of the eyelid. Dot eyeliner in a rounded arch at the base of lashes. Underline from outer corner to center, just below outside of pupil. Apply mascara to entire upper lashes.

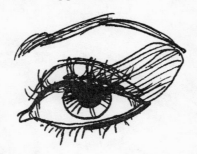

TO WIDEN CLOSE-SET EYES

Accent outer corners from center of the lids with a deeper shade eyeshadow, extending it to the end of the brows gradually fading out the color as it nears them. Use a light shade at the inside corners, blending it into the deeper shade. Use a natural tone concealer or highlighter in the corners at the bridge of the nose. (This adds width to this area.) Slightly extend your eyeliner past the outside corners of the eyes, and stop at the center of the lids over the pupils. Apply mascara only on outer lashes where it may be used heavily. Omit mascara on lower lashes.

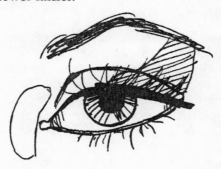

TO BRING WIDE-SET EYES IN CLOSER

Use a darker shade of eyeshadow on outer third of eyelids and extend it up to the brows gradually fading out the color as it nears them. Apply lighter shade of shadow to the inner two-thirds of the lids and extend it up to the brows blending it into the darker one-third portion. Line the eyes all the way to (but not into) the inner corners with eyeliner, avoiding it at the outer corner by ¼ inch. Concentrate mascara on center lashes only.

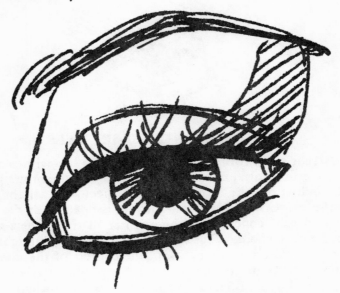

TO ENHANCE "LARGE" WIDE-SET EYES AND BRING THEM CLOSER TOGETHER

Apply soft subdued eyeshadow shades of blue, green, etc., to inner two-thirds of lids and area above, extending to the brows. Repeat the same shade on outer one-third just under the lower lids—smudge with cotton swab. Use taupe or light brown on outer one-third of eyelids to the brows and blend into the subdued shade making sure there is no line of demarcation. (Narrowing the bridge of nose with contour shading is a further enhancer, see page 199.) Apply eyeliner on eyelids to inside corners avoiding outer corners by ¼ inch.

Line lower lids not quite to inside corners. Mascara all of upper lashes concentrating mostly on center lashes. Lightly mascara lower lashes (optional).

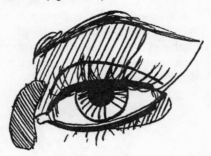

TO DRAMATIZE LIGHT-COLORED EYES
NEEDING MORE DEPTH

Apply smoky shade of eyeshadow (a smoky blue if your eyes are light blue, smoky green if eyes are light green, or smoky grey if eyes are light grey, etc.,) all around the eyes. Start on the eyelids, extending it to the upper lids, and continuing under the eyes smudging the color with cotton swab and stopping well short of inside corners. Use light beige eyeshadow up to the brow line to complete the upper lid area, blending into the smoky color so there are no lines of demarcation. Apply the narrowest line of offblack eyeliner to upper and lower eyelids, again stopping short of inside corners (see pages 203–204 for technique). Mascara upper and lower lashes but not too thickly. Length is more important than density to bring out the beautiful color of your eyes.

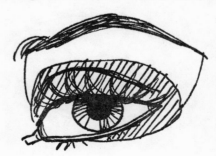

TO ELONGATE ROUND EYES

Use a subdued shade of taupe or light brown eyeshadow over the outer half of the eyelids to the crease. Follow the outer half of the crease-line in a darker brown. Use a light shade of shadow to the brows, extending it outward at the outer corners of the eyes. Use eyeliner from the center of the lids, slightly past outer corners. Concentrate mascara on upper outer lashes.

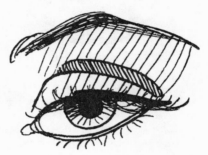

TO MINIMIZE PROTRUDING ROUND EYES

Use dark smoky shade of eyeshadow over entire eyelids from inner corners to slightly past outer corners. Use dark brown or offblack crayon or pencil and gently line the inside rims of upper and lower lids to diminish the whites of the eyes which make them look popped (Note: see pages 204–205). Use mascara lightly concentrating most on upper outer lashes.

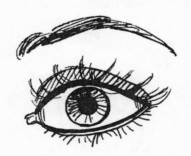

TO OPEN UP SQUINTY EYES OR
NARROW EYES

Use a light shade of eyeshadow and apply it high and center on the lids. Line outer half of upper lids only to make them appear rounder. Omit underlining except for a very slight line at the outside corners (optional). Apply mascara only to the center of upper lashes, heavily.

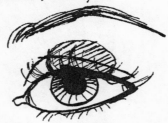

TO ELONGATE HORIZONTALLY
NARROW EYES

Use a light eyeshadow (pale taupe) at the center of the eyelids from lashline to crease. Use a deeper shade (medium taupe) on the inside corners of the lids blending into the light center shade. Use a still deeper hue (deep taupe) on outside corners of the lids extending it beyond the outer corners. Again blend this shade into the light center shade but maintain original placement for all three hues. (This concept may be used with any color eyeshadow using three hues of the same shade.) Apply eyeliner in an exceptionally thin ribbon across the eyelids (see pages 203–204 for technique). Concentrate mascara mostly on outer lashes. Underlining is optional when using suggested shades but if using colored eyeshadow, use the deepest shade as an underliner to the outside of the iris.

TO DIMINISH PROMINENT LIDS

Use brown or grey eyeshadow over the entire lids. Use a light beige tone from the crease on the upper lid to the brow. Apply eyeliner in a slightly heavier ribbon across entire eye and use a somewhat heavier application of mascara.

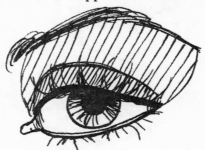

TO SHAPE ALREADY WELL-PROPORTIONED "LARGE" EYES

Apply eyeshadow in smoky shades of taupe, brown, grey, or soft subdued shades of blue, green, etc., to the entire eyelids. Blend carefully to fade out the color as it approaches the brows. (A dash of a still deeper shade may be shaded over the browbone, blended together.) Use deep brown or charcoal grey in the creases. Apply eyeliner in a not-too-thin ribbon (but also not too thick) across entire lids following the natural curve. Use dark brown or black crayon or pencil and gently line the inside rims of the lower lashes avoiding the inside of corners. (Note: see pages 204–205) . Apply mascara in generous doses to upper and lower lashes, separating so they do not look clumped together.

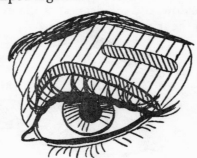

TO PICK UP DROOPY, SLEEPY LOOKING EYES

Apply smoky shade of eyeshadow (taupes, browns, grey, etc.) to the center of the eyelids very close to the lashes. At the outer corners extend the color upward. Use eyeliner from the center of the eyelids gradually widening the line and ending with a slightly upward tilt (a modified wing). Then continue the line just under the lower lashes terminating at the center of the eye. Curl the lashes with an eyelash curler and use mascara lightly on both upper and lower lashes.

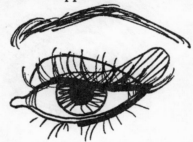

TO CONTOUR SLANTED EYES

Apply brighter shades of eyeshadow (blues, greens, etc.) to the center of the eyelids and extend the color upward at the outer corners. Use a light neutral shade over the rest of the eyelids. Extend it to the upper lids to soften the hard edges of the brighter shade but maintain its original outline. Use eyeliner from the center of the eyelids ending with a slightly upward tilt (a modified wing that is not overly oriental), and continue the line just under the lower lashes, terminating at the center of the eye. Concentrate mascara on outer lashes (lower lashes optional).

TO DISGUISE HEAVY FOLDS OVER THE
OUTER HALF OF UPPER LIDS

Use a light eyeshadow on the inner portion of the eyelids and under the brows. Use a dark smoky shade on the outer half of the lids and extend it to the brow line. Carefully blend, fading one shade into the other but maintain its original placement. Use liner and mascara only on the outer half of the lids.

TO DISGUISE OVERHANGING UPPER LIDS

Use a light neutral eyeshadow over the eyelids and a smoky brown or grey shadow starting from the upper side of the overhang to just above its lower edge. Repeat the lighter shade just under the brows. Blend well so that each shade fades into the other but maintain its original placement. Omit liner and use mascara heavily on upper lashes curling them as much as possible, so that lashes further throw natural shadows on the overhanging upper lids. Use mascara very lightly on lower lashes (optional) .

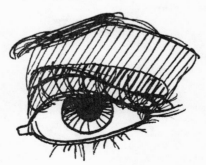

TO REDUCE BULGES BELOW THE BROWS

Shade bulging areas with brown or grey eyeshadow. Then use a light shade (light blue or green) near the lashes only. (Color near the lashes distracts the bulges.) Then use a dark eyeliner on both upper and lower lids from outside corner to center of lids. Underlining in blue is optional. Apply mascara only to outer half of upper and lower lashes.

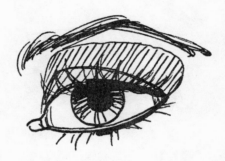

TO DISGUISE OLDER LOOKING EYES

Use a deep smoky tone eyeshadow and apply it on the upper lids over the creases of the normal lids. Blend close to the brows gradually fading out the color as it nears them. Omit underlining. Apply mascara only to the center of upper lashes, heavily.

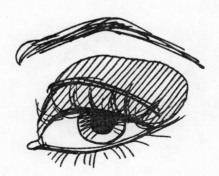

TO MAKE EYELIDS MORE PROMINENT

Use white or offwhite eyeshadow over entire lids. Line the upper portion of the crease with deep brown. Use eyeliner in an exceptionally thin ribbon across the eyelids (see pages 203–204 for technique) . Use mascara sparingly.

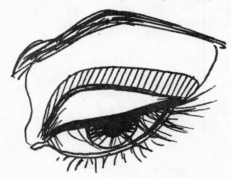

TO CONTOUR SOMEWHAT FLAT LIDS
FOR A ROUNDER LOOK

Use a light eyeshadow (pale peach is good in this instance) at the center of the eyelids. Use any deeper shade on the inside and outside corners of the lids blending into the light center shade. (Heaviest concentration of color should border the light centered area and fade off to the corners.) Use a deep brown or any dark shade in the crease. Dot eyeliner in a rounded arch at the base of the lashes. Underlining is optional. Mascara all of the upper lashes.

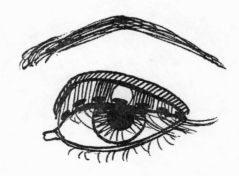

TO LIGHTEN DARK EYELIDS AND
CORRECT CORNER SHADOWS

Use white, offwhite, or beige eyeshadow or highlighter or natural shade of concealer over the entire lids, extending it into the corner at the bridge of nose. Shade a tiny bit of taupe or brown shadow at the corners on sides of nose where it best contours the bridge in proportion to the eyes and vice versa. (This is not the same location where the original dark shadow existed. If you find it is, then you do not require this improvement.) Smudge the spot with a cotton swab or sponge applicator softening it so there are no lines of demarcation. Proceed with eye makeup according to the shape of your eyes.

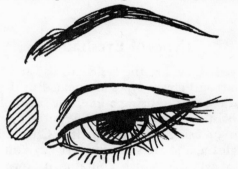

TO REDUCE PUFFINESS UNDER THE EYES

Use offwhite eyeshadow from the crease of the eyelids to the brows. Emphasis is put on eyeliner to contour the eyelids to their best proportions according to the shape of the eyes. Use lots of mascara on upper lashes only. (Also see pages 67 and 137.)

EYESHADOW

The play of shadows falling on a given object are never one shade alone. They are variations and gradations of shades and the fall of light on them is what makes the object look interesting. This is especially true of eyeshadow. The use of only one bright shade of eyeshadow on the lids is harsh, unnatural and obscures the beauty of the eyes. For most shapes of eyes (the exceptions are noted in the previous illustrations), the blending of two or three shades of eyeshadow produces a subtle, natural effect that enhances eye color and shape. *Eyeshadow should do just that—* shadow the eyes—not obscure them with a flat mask of any one color.

Types of Eyeshadow

Powdered eyeshadows are the easiest to use and are the longest wearing. Crayons and cream types are next. But if you use cream, try to get into the habit of using a fine, flat bristle brush to apply it (sable with bristles about $1/4$-inch wide is the best). The results are so superior to using your fingertips. Creams do give more highlight and gleam, and are good for very dry skin. Or try a flowing cream in a cylinder which contains its own applicator or built-in brush. Coloring pencils (crayons) glide on smoother and blend easier if you first use an eyeshadow base. Crayon, liquid, or tubestick eyeshadows require holding (not stretching) the eyelids taut in order to assure a fine blending of the color.

For daytime I suggest eyeshadow shades of dark and light neutrals—smoky taupes and browns to give depth and definition or shades of grey. And pale beige to white for highlighting, or soft shades of pink or peach.

White and offwhite (including any pale shade in the category of cream, buff, bone, sand, or beige) are used to highlight the eyelids, to enlarge the eyes, or to bring out deep-set eyes, or to highlight other areas that need to be contrasted by darker shades. It is also used sparingly just below the eyebrows to give them more definition. It opens up the eyes and plays up or simulates good bone structure. Also, whites, when used underneath other shades, soften their tones. Pink or peach may be used to accent the browbone or lid but must be applied in small doses and be blended well to appear natural. (If your complexion leans toward the ruddy, avoid the latter two shades altogether.)

Shades of brown, taupe, grey, and violet are used to diminish protruding contours, such as contouring the bone area with a darker shade to correct bone structure. These shades are also used to correct protruding eyes or eyelids that are larger than normal size in relation to the face.

In addition to the neutral tones I have suggested for everyday wear, eyeshadow colors may be chosen to enhance the eye color itself, or by matching or contrasting it. They may also be chosen to complement the garment you intend to wear. When you can find wardrobes of colors already assembled for your convenience by the manufacturer, they are usually the best buys.

Frosted or luminous shades in stronger colors are most effective for evening wear but should be confined to evening alone. The silver, gold, and platinum shadows are very dramatic touches for evening or gala occasions.

If you have difficulty in applying any eye makeup because of constant or excessive blinking, open your mouth to a wide "O." This will tense the muscles of the face and enable you to apply the various techniques over a longer period of time without blinking, thereby speeding up the application of all your eye makeup. This is particularly helpful when applying false eyelashes.

When making up your eyes, look down into your magnifying mirror. The top should be tilted slightly toward you if you are sitting. Tilt the top of the mirror back slightly if you are standing while you are making up. Then step back two to four feet to check the overall effect in a regular mirror.

Shading and Blending Color Lesson

The principle of light and dark is again reflected in these techniques of applying eyeshadow. (Remember, the principle of *all* makeup is light and dark.) This also carries through when you wish to use colors. When you know how to apply the neutral shades I have suggested for everyday use, then you will use the same principle with more vivid colors for evening.

We'll use green for an example:

WE'LL USE GREEN FOR AN EXAMPLE:

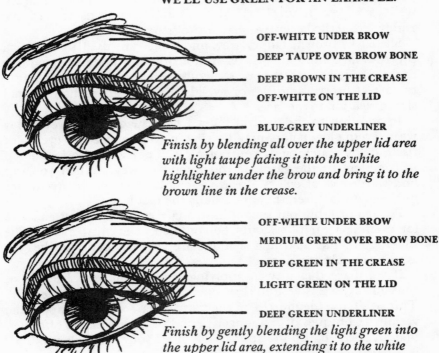

OFF-WHITE UNDER BROW

DEEP TAUPE OVER BROW BONE

DEEP BROWN IN THE CREASE

OFF-WHITE ON THE LID

BLUE-GREY UNDERLINER

Finish by blending all over the upper lid area with light taupe fading it into the white highlighter under the brow and bring it to the brown line in the crease.

OFF-WHITE UNDER BROW

MEDIUM GREEN OVER BROW BONE

DEEP GREEN IN THE CREASE

LIGHT GREEN ON THE LID

DEEP GREEN UNDERLINER

Finish by gently blending the light green into the upper lid area, extending it to the white highlighter under the brows and bringing it to the deep green or brown in the crease.

Allow the powdered type of eyeshadow to set for a moment and then whisk away any excess before you apply your eyeliner. To hold the cream or crayon types better, lightly dust on translucent powder over the eyelids. Later you can touch them lightly with a cotton ball moistened in cool water and squeezed out almost dry (optional).

For a different effect try two textures—powder on the lids, cream on the browbone, or vice versa. Apply any eyeshadow with feather-light strokes, blending the color with the applicator or brush, either spreading, sweeping, or drawing (see pages 8–9) . Your touch should always be featherlike. It is important to use eye makeup in the proper sequence. Start at the top and work down. Shadows, eyeliner, mascara, or false lashes and then mascara. Sounds like a lot but it actually isn't. There is no need to be timid, there is simply need to use them deftly. Your eyeshadow will virtually last all day when properly applied.

EYELINER

The next step is eyeliner. Use liquid, cake with water, crayon or pencil, or automatic type in cylinders with their own built-in brushes, or even dark shades of powdered eyeshadow.

Since I was virtually one of the first to mass market eye makeup, and first with the liquid eyeliner (the forerunner of all types of modern eyeliners), I was obliged to instruct the beauty advisors and cosmeticians through their schools throughout the country, so that they in turn could instruct you. And through various instruction booklets packaged with products and other media about the application of eye makeup, I came directly into your home with instructions that you are probably using. I would now like to reverse a procedure that I started many years ago and perhaps you are still using today. Through repeated testing and on practically all eye shapes, I find that this method is easier and the results are better and more natural looking, especially since the exaggerated upturned wings of the 1960s passed into oblivion and now look so foolish.* (Since history always repeats itself they will probably see a future revival, but for now the dark, smudged look is in and is so much softer looking.)

Originally, I instructed women to hold the eyelids taut (somehow during the course of the years, it became *s t r e t c h* the eyelids taut—and that should also be added to your "no-no" list) and draw the liner from the inside corner to the outside corner. You may be well accustomed to this procedure and have mastered it very well, but if you try the one I now suggest, I think you will like it.

It is simply to start at the *outside corner* of the eye and draw the line *inward*, without holding the eyelid taut or using your other hand in any way. This technique will permit you to draw a thinner line and you will be less likely to draw it all the way into the inner corner. Actually, you can stop anywhere along the way. I think you will find it not only easier, but faster. The results certainly look more natural. You can then use the blue underliner

---

* There are some otherwise smart looking women who are still wearing this exaggerated look. I would very much like to impress upon them how passé it really is. If this style is good for your eye shape (and there are some contours for which it is used as a corrective), at least modify it. There is no need to look dated when a mere modification will make you look fashionable.

—either pencil, powder, liquid, or crayon—from the same starting point, but please don't go to the inner corners unless you have wide-set eyes.

Another technique you might try in order to arrive at a super-thin line is to first brush the lashes downward with mascara, then apply your eyeliner, and then apply mascara brushing the lashes upward.

Shades for Eyelining

Jet black should be reserved for evening wear when one uses black mascara, unless you are a dramatic brunette type. Offblack, black-brown, deep browns, medium browns, plums, taupes, or charcoal grey are better for daytime. A good effect for just a hint of color is to use a thin ribbon of green, blue, or turquoise, etc., just above the basic eyeliner. Colors should be applied first so that your basic shade is as close as possible to the roots of the lashes.

If you want the smudged look, which is fashionable at the moment and really makes the eyes look very sensuous and pretty, don't try to smudge liquid eyeliner, it will only make a mess. Use either pencil or powdered eyeshadow, using a fine, short bristle eyeliner brush. You can smudge the penciled line with your little finger or blur it with a cotton swab. The powder gives it to you automatically. Deep burgundies, dark grey, offblack and brown powdered eyeshadows work best and are the quickest and easiest product to achieve this look.

Underlining the Eyes

A thick jet-black line drawn into the inside corners on the lower lashes is a mistake. It closes the eyes in and makes them look smaller and what's worse, cold and harsh.

In addition, black or any other color eyeliner should not be placed on the lower *inner* rims of the eyes. The exception being if you have huge eyes and want to reduce their apparent size. Even this is frowned upon by the American Medical Association, for it can lead to various eye problems, particularly of the conjunctiva (the membrane lining the lids and covering the exposed surface of the eyeballs) . So be wary, even though I have suggested that women with certain eye shapes (specifically, protruding round eyes and well-proportioned "large" eyes) use this technique in order to make their eyes look their utmost, then lining the inner rim does become the necessary method. But if you have one of these eye shapes and you have a tendency toward any eye problems, omit lining the inner rim—it just isn't worth the risk.

For the rest of us who don't have any eye problems and who don't want to encourage them, underlining with any type of eyeliner should be on the skin surface just under the lower lashes. Stop where the inner eyelashes do not normally grow to avoid going into the corners of the eyes.

Eyeliner and False Eyelashes

Apply the liner to your eyelids first, and then touch up after the false lashes have been applied—if it is required. I know many women like to apply their supplemental lashes first and then use the liner, but this usually results in the line becoming too thick. This is because the shadow cast by the lashes themselves is obstructing the view and forcing you to use a heavier hand, when what you need is a steadier hand. *Stop!* It seems you're always told to use a steady hand but no one seems to bother to tell you how to do it. There are several methods, such as resting your elbow on the table surface in front of you, or steadying your little finger on your cheek, but I like this one best. Simply, lightly hold the wrist of your applying hand with the other hand. The fingers

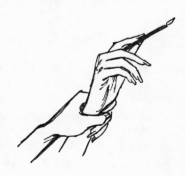

should close on the inside of the wrist of the applying hand. Try it my way for both of these techniques—I'm sure you'll find it easier.

Types of Eyeliners and Removers

Eyeliners are available in liquid, pencil, crayon, powder, and automatic cylinders with brushes. Some are waterproof. They are removed with a solvent such as mineral oil or similar oils which are also found in most facial cleansing creams and lotions. Or you may prefer special eye makeup removers and/or pads. Be sure to use your eyewash to remove all traces of residue (see page 57) for nothing is as soothing to your eyes as an isotonic solution.

The Care of Your Brushes

The care of your brushes is simple. They usually require nothing more than wiping away any excess with a tissue and tapering the bristles with your fingertips. On occasion you may dip them into 70 percent alcohol to cleanse and then reshape them with your fingers. Good bristle brushes are a fine investment (I'm still using the same ones I've had for at least twenty years). For brushes with nylon bristles, wash them in soap and water.

EYELASHES

Eyelash Curlers

If you use an eyelash curler (a practice many of us never gave up since our teens), employ it after your eyeliner and before mascara. Place the curler on the base of the lashes and while holding it in a stationary position, squeeze the handle several times so that it opens and closes on the lashes. Curling your lashes not only gives them deeper emphasis and curliness, but will cause the lashes to cast shadows on the eyelids instead of the eyes themselves. This also opens up the appearance of the eyes. (Women with overhanging upper lids will find this extremely advantageous.)

Eyelash curlers will not break your eyelashes unless the rubber insert is hard, worn down, or missing. The curlers are made to accommodate refillable rubber cushion inserts. While they are long lasting, it is wise to keep an extra refill on hand so you can quickly snap it in when replacement becomes necessary.

Care of Your Eyelashes

Almost all women have the normal number of eyelashes—approximately 75 to 100 hairs on each of her upper eyelids and 25 to 40 on the lower lids. There is no external cream or lotion that can either make them grow longer or more dense. But you can use a conditioner to make the lashes silkier and to keep them from becoming brittle, especially if you do not ordinarily wear mascara which contains conditioners.

While 75 to 100 upper eyelashes may seem like a lot of hairs, remember you normally lose about 100 hairs each day from your head. This is considered an infinitesimal amount considering that, on the average, you have between 100,000 and 200,000 hairs on your head, and they are constantly being replaced as they fall out or break off. Eyelashes too, are gradually shed and replaced every two to three months.

The shampoos we use all contain conditioning agents, and many of us use additional conditioners to maintain the beauty and health of our hair. Eyelashes deserve at least some of the same consideration. If you use mascara on a day-to-day basis, then your eyelashes are probably receiving enough conditioners although any extra certainly won't hurt. But if you do not wear mascara, then you might consider a conditioner for your lashes (the same conditioner can also be used on eyebrows) which may be used day or night or both. These are available as a cream or an automatic roll-on applicator. They do not contain the dark coloring agents used in mascara, but will add luster while they silken and enhance your eyelashes.

In answer to a question that crops up every so often: "Will my eyelashes grow back if I lose them through some disorder or injury?" The answer is that it depends upon the individual damage. If the hair follicles remain intact and uninjured, the lashes will grow back, probably within two to three months when they would ordinarily replace themselves. If they do not grow back, false eyelashes are a far better choice than seeking eyelash implants which have been known to cause many eye problems.

Mascara

For most women, the automatic roll-on mascara with built-in brush is the easiest and most convenient to use. For some women, especially those who have very light or sparse lashes, it is preferable to start by applying mascara on the upper side of the lashes and brush them downward. (This also enables you to draw a super thin line with your eyeliner.) Then, apply upward from underneath, continuously twirling the handle between your fingers as you apply it to your lashes. For other types of mascara, brush upward with light lifting motions. Brushing both sides of the lashes gives them greater thickness. Apply mascara to one eye and then the other. Repeat applications in successive order if you wish to build. Two or three thin applications allowing the lashes to dry before the next application is always better than one thick coat. If they stick together, use a special eyelash comb or carefully use the point of a **Pick-A-Dent** (see page 210) to separate them. Always apply mascara from the roots to the tips holding the brush horizontal to the eye. Avoid getting the mascara onto the inside rim of the eyelid (upper or lower). This too may risk conjunctivitis. If you should happen to smudge it on the inner rim, you can easily remove it with a moistened cotton swab. Use either water or sterile eye drops, making sure there are no loose cotton fibers. If you find it difficult to apply mascara to the lashes of your lower lids, try this: First sweep them upward from underneath with the brush, then sideways using the tip of the brush, then downward, separating and placing them correctly.

Types of Mascara

Mascara comes in many forms: Liquid in a bottle, cream in a tube, cake moistened with water, roll-on automatic applicator with brush (straight or spiral), comb, or a combination of brush and comb. They all separate and curl. Some mascaras have lash builders that have tiny filaments that cling to your own lashes, extending them by making them thicker and longer. Any of these may be a waterproof mascara, which holds fast and sees you through tears and rain. When using cake mascara, which requires wetting the brush with water (not saliva), make sure the brush is not overloaded. Look down into your mirror, the flat of the brush (sides of bristles) should be facing your face. Brush lightly with upward strokes.

MASCARA SHADE GUIDE
(Daytime)

Light blondes	Light brown, taupe
Medium to dark blondes	Light brown, medium brown
Brownettes	Medium brown, dark brown, black-brown
Brunettes	Dark brown, black-brown, charcoal grey, black
Light redheads	Light brown, taupe
Medium and dark redheads	Medium brown, taupe, charcoal grey, black-brown
Silver or Grey	Light brown, taupe, charcoal grey

(Black or midnight blue may be substituted for evening by everyone)

Supplemental Eyelashes

There always seems to be a new and easier method for applying false eyelashes, but I'll bet dollars to donuts that you'll find this one easiest and most effective. For those women who think they can't apply false eyelashes, you can attain what may have always appeared to be difficult.

Use a curved, scissor-handled tweezer (**Twissors** by Kurlash and

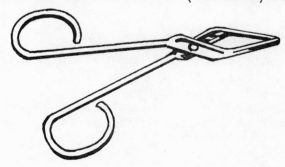

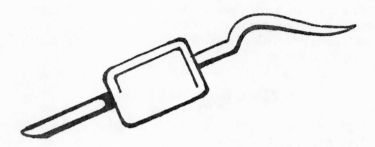

Revlon manufactures them). The curved design permits you better vision. You will also need a little plastic device called **Pick-A-Dent**. It is a small, curved, plastic gadget that comes in pretty colors and is used for the teeth (little did they dream!). It is purchased at your local drug store, usually in packages of four. This little device has many advantages over an ordinary toothpick which most women usually use for this purpose.

• It is colored, so you can find it easily (the toothpick always seems to get lost).

• The curved design allows you to see better and gives you more efficient control to apply the adhesive to the narrow band of the lashes.

• The center handle gives your fingers something more to grasp for better control.

• The straight end has a flat, tapered edge which is better to tap down the lash once you have applied it to your own, and it is safer than a toothpick.

• It is forever reusable and is cleaned merely by tissuing off and occasionally washing in soap and water.

The Technique

Put a drop of adhesive on a tissue (that's all you need) and then close the cap to the tube. Grasp the lash by the tips with the tweezer. Take the **Pick-A-Dent** and pick up a tiny amount of adhesive with the curved, pointed end. Apply adhesive to the back of the band, spreading thinly. Still holding the lash with the tweezer, *zoom-in* with the back of your hand facing the mirror and your closed fingers facing you. Land it right on top of your own lashes. Adjust, so that the lashband slides into the little groove at the root of your lashes.

First make sure the lashes extend no further out at the outside corners than your own lashes and preferably *within* one or two of your own. Then gently tap down with the flat part of the straight end of the **Pick-A-Dent.** In following this method, you will usually get them on just right, but always check from a profile angle with a hand mirror. (I still do even though I can apply them in ten seconds.) More important, observe from an overhead view to make sure the curve of the lashband is properly in place. Pinch together with your fingertips or use the tweezers in a position parallel to the eye. Now apply mascara, blending your own lashes and those you've supplemented together, but do not mascara all the way to the tips. That's it!

Lightly mascara the lower lashes from underneath. First sweep them upward, then sideways with the tip of the brush, then downward with the brush from over the top. Although I consider it quite unnecessary, some women like false bottom lashes (there are special ones made just for this purpose) to supplement their own lower lashes. If so, use the above described method for applying them.

Wearing supplemental lashes can become second nature if they are lightweight and not dense, and they have a very thin lashband. You won't even be aware that you are wearing them and neither will anyone else. They don't have to be too long or look false—just enough to make well defined eyes. Time alone thins and lightens our own eyelashes, and more mature women need mascara and/or lashes more than ever. But you don't want them to look contrived. Demi-lashes are just right for daytime. You can treat them as if they were your very own lashes. They are not that fragile. Women who try to make their lashes last indefinitely always look like they are wearing false eyelashes. They should be selected according to the method of applying mascara for individual eye shapes as described on pages 186 through 199.

Lightly apply mascara to your own eyelashes first, and then again apply mascara once the supplemented lashes are in place, to blend them together. Or you may just apply mascara to both lashes upon completion of their application.

Removing Supplemental Lashes

Remove lashes by carefully gripping one end of the lashband at the outer corner using your thumb and index finger and gently peel toward the inner corner. Peel adhesive off if you do not intend to treat them with a lash cleaner.

Some women complain that when they remove their lashes they are simultaneously pulling off their own lashes as well, or they say that they are afraid of breaking their own lashes. If you avoid the following pitfalls this will no longer be a problem.

• Using the above directions to remove, make sure to peel not only gently but slowly.

• Avoid using too much adhesive when applying the lashes to your own. For good adhesion they require only the thinnest coating.

• Do not apply lashes that have a gummed up adhesive coating left over from a previous wearing. Lashes should be cleaned of all debris.

• At night always thoroughly cleanse your eyes of old mascara which can cause eyelashes to break. The accumulation of debris and pollutants picked up during the day contributes to this. If you are a woman who likes to wear her mascara to bed (yes, there are some women who like to do this), apply a fresh application.

Manufacturers supply a good adhesive with the initial purchase of false eyelashes, but if you find you have to buy it separately, buy a clear drying eyelash adhesive that is of surgical quality.

TYPES OF FALSE EYELASHES
(Supplemental)

Demi	For everyday wear—adds fullness from center of the eyelids to the outer corners.
Spaced	Full length, but spaced to supplement your own lashes and to open up small or deep-set eyes.
Natural	Full length basic eyelashes
Full	More lush, better for evening, but good on some women for daywear.
Shaggy	Long and full with criss-cross hairs. Should be reserved for very large eyes or for evening wear only.
Individual	Small sections of two or three hairs. Good for adding fullness where it is wanted.

Caring for Your Supplemental Eyelashes

There is one personal practice I would like to pass on to you. Although it is not necessarily right for everyone, it is very convenient for some. Use it if you think it suits your style.

I have a wardrobe of nine pairs of eyelashes—one for every day of the week, one for emergency, and a special, more glamorous pair for special occasions. I use very natural mini-lashes and I apply them daily by blending them into my own lashes with mascara, not too much, I don't want a heavy mascara-ed look for daytime. Naturally, when I remove them at night they are soiled with adhesive, old mascara, plus dirt, grime, and pollutants, picked up from the day's activities. Frankly, I cannot be bothered to peel the adhesive and clean them every night, so I just put them into a small container reserved for this purpose. Once a week (during my own special time) I pour a chemical lash cleaner into the same container to let them soak for a few minutes, then I take the special lash brush (supplied in the package) and clean them all at once. I place them one at a time on a tissue and brush the dirt and old adhesive off the lash right onto the tissue—the debris adheres to the tissue as I keep moving the false lash to a clean spot on it, until the lash is entirely clean. As I complete each lash, I lay it out on a clean tissue to absorb any excess cleaner. When I'm finished cleaning, I sort them into pairs and put them back on their original platform in the individual boxes. (This still retains the sticky strip on which the lashes came and keeps them flexed for proper contour.) There is no need to curl or fuss with them any further. They are like new and are clean and ready for the following week.

Of course, you really don't need nine pairs to work with. You could use four pairs and apply the same cleaning procedure twice a week. If you are the type who likes to wash her pantyhose every night, you may like to care for your lashes daily, too.

False Eyelashes that Really Look False

Many false eyelashes are too wide, too big, too long, and distinctly phony looking. Lashes that are sparse, lightweight, have a very thin band, are pre-trimmed and need only to be adjusted in width are a better choice any day of the week. False eyelashes should supplement your own lashes and not look like you're wearing phonies.

However, if it is necessary to alter your false eyelashes—and in many cases it is a must because of the way many are manufactured, here's how to adjust them.

Use a safety razor (one edge) and place the lashes on a flat cutting surface. (A magazine may be used to protect the underlying surface.) Place a sheet of white paper on top so that you can easily see what you are cutting.

Place the lashes upside down. Shorten their length to fit your eye. Slice off the end that would go on the outside corner of your eye. Check and adjust. Do the same for the other lash. Cut the individual hairs to a length you think would look most natural on you. Using a rocking, back and forth motion with the razor blade, slice off the tips of 2 or 3 hairs at a time and continue around, maintaining the original curve of the lash. Shape the other lash as closely as possible to the first.

If you are anything less than thrilled with the outcome, then next time buy lashes already trimmed and shaped to your liking. The only time you ought to cut or trim these yourself is when they become old and a bit ragged. Then snip off the bad ends on either side and use them for mini-lashes or cut them up and use them individually.

Individual Supplemental Eyelashes

Individual lashes are still another alternative. They are especially good for those eye shapes that require mascara concentrated in certain areas (refer to your eye shape, pages 186 to 199). Apply them using a scissor-handled tweezer and dip the tip of the lash into a large drop of adhesive placed on a folded tissue. Use only the tiniest amount of adhesive, blotting off any excess onto the tissue before applying to your eye. Rest it at the base of your own lashes and gently press together with the tweezer. A light coating of mascara may be used to blend them together. However, these lashes are very effective without mascara. Use only regular eyelash adhesive which is of surgical quality. The more permanent type of glue usually supplied with these kinds of commercial, ready-made lashes can make your own lashes break. The individual lashes won't last for more than a day with the surgical type adhesive, but who wants to risk shorter lashes than we already have?

A WORD OF CAUTION

Please remember that eyelid tissue is thin and delicate, the thinnest skin of your entire body. If you are a novice and at first you experience some difficulty in applying eye makup, or the effect is too much for you (it shouldn't be if you use the shades I've suggested), don't cleanse it off more than once. Repeated cleansing of eye makeup within a short period of time will irritate this delicate area and cause your eyes to tear or sting and become red. This might cause you to think that you are allergic to the product. Please believe me, it is the repeated cleansings and re-applications, and most likely not the product, that cause the irritation.

GOOD MAKEUP AND PRECIOUS TIME

How long does it take to apply makeup? Is that what you're thinking? Well, certainly applying eye makeup takes longer than the rest but I do not believe in setting a time limit for each individual procedure. Everyone works at a different pace, no matter what one might be working at. One woman might charge through her housework in the morning while another dawdles, and still they will both achieve the same degree of cleanliness. By the same token, one woman is capable of applying her entire makeup including false eyelashes in six or seven minutes while another woman needs twenty-five or thirty minutes, even though they will both achieve the same degree of expertise. I would say the average would be fifteen to twenty minutes for a complete makeup. Just keep in mind though, that the more often you wear a complete makeup, the quicker and more adept you become. Even the busiest woman can manage fifteen or twenty minutes each day for her own face. If you're not worth it, who is?

EYEGLASSES

For women with normal vision between the ages of 30 and 45, a five year eye check-up is usually adequate. (Of course, there are always the exceptions—women who experience sudden or acute symptoms, or the woman who one day realizes that she can't thread a needle. Don't hesitate. Phone for an appointment.)

After the age of forty-five everyone should have a "thorough" yearly check-up with an ophthalmologist*—a physician who specializes in eye care—because eyes change, gradually declining in their focusing ability. Women who have never worn glasses before find that they need reading glasses and this is common in at least 80 percent of this age group.

Women who have previously worn eyeglasses may find at around age 45 that they require glasses for near and distance vision. Bifocals with the distinct segment line between the two different lenses are not usually appealing to nor attractive on most women. While switching from distance to reading glasses may be a nuisance, it is preferable. However, new lenses are now available that are either seamless to the viewer (but not the wearer) or "progressive" allowing for a gradual change of focus with no outwardly visible lines.

Eye makeup is so important to the appearance of women who constantly need to wear eyeglasses. Nearsighted (*myopic*) women may use brighter, more intense colors of eyeshadow (the lenses tend to obscure or decrease the size of the eyes), but these shades should take all factors into consideration and should be especially flattering to the eyes, frames, and color of clothing. Farsighted (*presbyopic*) women whose corrective lenses tend to magnify the eyes should avoid bright colored eyeshadow altogether as the results look much too theatrical. The neutrals and smokey tones I have suggested are best for all occasions. A slight touch of lipgloss or a bit of blush just above the brows will give the eyes more sparkle. And remember, keep the natural brow line where it belongs, even though the frames may be higher. Of course, lenses should always be sparkling clean, not only for good vision but also to let your viewers see the beauty of your eyes.

If you wear supplemental eyelashes, be sure to wear them at the time of your eye examination, so that any new prescription will take their length into consideration and accommodate a slight

---

* While an optometrist (O.D.) is also good for this age group, he is limited to prescribing glasses and exercises. If he detects any eye disease he will have to refer you to an ophthalmologist (M.D.). An ophthalmologist has the full range of diagnostic equipment and experience to detect all symptoms of eye disease and prescribe any and all medical treatment.

extra curvature that might be required for the lenses. And, when you visit your optician for new glasses, it is always wise to wear eye makeup so that the two can be coordinated.

If you find it difficult to make up your eyes because you need your glasses, you might consult your optician about frames with specially hinged lenses. These glasses permit you the vision of one eye while you make up the other. It's a great boon for those who need it—and even better when used in conjunction with a magnifying mirror.

Women who need to work very close to their mirrors should select cosmetic tools with very short handles. When this is not possible, as in the case of eyebrow or lip pencils, choose thin wooden ones that can be broken in half and sharpened.

Women who are myopic and wear contact lenses have to be extremely careful when applying makeup. To eliminate the possibility of clouding the lenses, you should apply all preparation and foundation makeup first and insert the contacts just before applying your eye makeup. At this point, you must be very careful not to get any eye makeup into the eye, since it will cause discomfort and cloud the lenses. Always wash your hands and rinse them thoroughly before inserting the contacts to make sure they do not have any traces of makeup or soap residue, which will also cloud the lenses. And should you get some eye makeup into the eye, put a few drops of saline solution on a cotton swab (make sure to wet it *thoroughly* so there are no loose fibers), and gently lift the debris *only from the corner* of the eye. However, if the matter is in the eye itself, you will have to remove the contact and recleanse. When inserting and removing contacts, be very careful about stretching or pulling at the delicate skin around the eyes, and don't rub. These manipulations cause wrinkles and contribute to the ones you may already have. Be gentle and treat your eyes tenderly.

Eyeglasses and Your Face Shape

Today eyeglasses are so imaginatively designed that I think they are more of a fashion asset than the liability Dorothy Parker once noted them for (circa 1932). Time and fashion designers have proven her wrong! Men *do* make passes at *we* girls who wear glasses (the italics mine). But it is vitally important to select colors of frames to harmonize with your hair and eyebrows, and the shape should flatter your features as well as your face shape. The following guide is keyed for your face shape—you'll have to take into consideration your individual features, keeping in mind that eye makeup shades should be coordinated to the frame's color. And for evening wear, regardless of your coloring, nothing is as flattering as the glint of a thin rim of a gold or silver frame.

Oval	The world of eyeglasses may be of your choosing, taking into account your special features, but the frames should be as wide or slightly wider than the broadest part of your face.
Round	The frames should be moderately deep and slightly wider than your cheeks, the lower edge of the frame arching in an upward curve such as the new themes on the old harlequin shape. Square, rectangular, octagonal shapes can also be effective. Avoid frames that are too round.
Square	The frames should be wider than the broadest part of your jawline with a curved lower edge and an arched upper. Large size frames look well on you. Avoid square shapes and straight lines.
Heart-Shaped	The frames should be short vertically and extend to the hairline at the temples with a full lower edge suggesting a downward line. Avoid round shapes.
Diamond-Shaped	The frames should be as narrow or slightly narrower than the top part of your cheeks. There are many new shapes that you can wear effectively, but avoid a highly arched bridge.
Long, Oblong, or Inverted Triangle	The frames should be deep and as wide as the broadest part of your cheeks. Octagonal shapes will add

	width to a narrow forehead. Oval shapes are good for emphasizing width of the entire face.
Triangular	The upper part of the frames should be wider than the broadest points of your jawline and the frame's lower edge should be narrower, curving upward. Oval, square, or rectangular shapes are good but the latter should be selected avoiding harsh lines.

Sunglasses

Sunglasses are not only a fashion accessory used to protect our eyes from the sun in the summer, but a protective covering from the pollution and glare we are subject to throughout the year. To a large degree they prevent the inevitable squinting that would otherwise be our natural reflex. (Squinting is one of the worst causes of premature lines and wrinkles around the eyes, and accentuates the ones already there.) We need all the help we can get to retard this predisposition. The lenses should be of fine optical quality to prevent distortion. For bright sunlight and glare, grey or green lenses offer the best protection. The frames can be as dramatic or as simple as you like. The shape of sunglasses should also be coordinated to your face shape. Select a larger or heavier framed version of the shapes outlined in the preceding section.

However, if you wear glasses while driving, make sure that the temples (side pieces) are not too thick or in line with the pupils of your eyes. The side pieces should be higher or lower than the level of your pupils so as not to obstruct your peripheral vision. Some of those designer glasses with dramatically curved side pieces really have practical value for they eliminate this problem.

A suggested guide for the frame's color according to your individual coloring is provided below:

COLOR GUIDE FOR FRAMES OF SUNGLASSES

Blondes with fair complexions	Soft pastels, light tortoise tones

Blondes with medium to dark complexions	Cool blues, silvery striated colors, medium tortoise tones
Brownettes or brunettes with light complexions	Pastels, striated colors, tortoise tones, black
Brownettes or brunettes with medium to dark complexions	Cool whites, dark ambers, dark tortoise tones
Redheads	Smoky greys, greens, tortoise tones, black
Grey or white	Soft pastels, silvery blue tones
Black hair and skin	Pastels and high-intensity colors (purples, pinks, corals)

Lipstick Was Born in America in the 20th Century

Lipstick is every woman's favorite cosmetic. It is also a significant part of woman's history.

It was 1914 when tinted powder, rouge, and rouging the lips became the sudden excitement among the upper classes and for the few other women who could afford them. But, it was as early as 1886 that Harriet Hubbard Ayer predicted that women would be using tinted cosmetics in the future. After 1914 some of the smaller cosmetic companies attempted to make these new products more affordable to the young factory girls of the era. In 1915 the metal container had been invented so lipsticks (in their present form) could be mass produced, therefore driving down their prices. But still, because most middle class women had no money of their own they could not partake of the new social and fashion cosmetic trend.

Then the first World War came and while America remained neutral between August 1914 and March 1917, production of our own materials was cut back for the war effort for we were sending supplies and money to Britain and France long before we sent our boys over. In April 1917 America officially entered into the war and of course it was over for both America and Europe in November 1918. The moviegoers of 1918 saw Theda Bara wearing mascara and lipstick, as well as face powder and colored eye shadow and although the motion pictures of the time were not in color, women quickly grasped the concept of shading their eyes and wearing all the cosmetics together. By 1919 with the weary war over, American women were psychologically ready for the advent of makeup as a complete concept. They had been previously conditioned to single products, though of short duration and on a discriminated basis.

During the war years, class distinctions reversed as to the use and non-use of makeup. The upper class reverted to non-use and the middle and lower classes took it over, to the disapproval of their families and employers. For the first time, women were emancipated, for they were working and had money to spend on themselves. Cosmetics were considerably cheaper at that time. They were available in the chain stores that cultivated and catered to working women. Indeed the chain stores themselves were just coming into their own.

The roaring 20s blossomed with the flapper, and lipstick was truly born for all American women. European women* did not follow suit at first but within a few years the use of lipstick also became their way of life. European companies were now coming into existence and they showed their own brand of chic as they still do. It was a glamorous American era with F. Scott Fitzgerald portraying women to his readers as innocent but scandalous figures.

After the 1920s, cosmetics on a large scale died out again. The 1930s were conservative—they had to be, due to the Great Depression, although makeup did not entirely disappear from the scene. There were still some very rich people and wealthy women bought expensive products for they were once again exclusively in the province of the rich. Lipstick remained the darling of the less fortunate, for when a woman could not afford frivolities for herself, somehow she managed to buy herself a lipstick to lift up her spirits in a depressed world. This will probably always hold true for even in times of recession, cosmetic sales and therefore their stocks go up.

Even before the Great Depression, such giants as Elizabeth Ar-

* French women were the exception. With their usual fashion awareness they leaped on the bandwagon at the outset.

den and Helena Rubinstein had made their marks with treatment lines. American women were eagerly awaiting the return of the day when they could again afford their beloved cosmetics.

In 1932 Charles Revson created Revlon (along with his brothers and a man named Charles Lachman; the "L" in Revlon represented Mr. Lachman). The first Revlon product was nail polish (nail *"enamel"*—Charles Revson was adamant about this word and all his employees had to be careful not to use the word "polish," lest they lose their jobs). Lipsticks were to follow a few years later and matching lips and fingertips became the rage. Now the movies were having a tremendous impact on American women. Every woman wanted to look glamorous.

Then came World War II. While cosmetic production was not halted because it was deemed morale boosting to the war effort, still production was cut back because many ingredients were not available. Thus we had the thick, heavy, dark lipsticks of the 1940s. After 1945, with the war over, American women were ready for something new and more colors became available. Variety was now the spice of life (heretofore only three basic colors, red, orange, and pink had existed and subtle shades of these were yet to come, along with the more sophisticated and evocative shade names such as "Fire and Ice").

Now, many new cosmetic companies were started with an eye to the lucrative profits. The older perfume houses also expanded their lines into color products. They, too, wanted to compete and fulfill the ever-increasing demands for more and more, both on the part of women and on the part of cosmetic companies.

By the late 1940s television was within the monetary reach of the average American family and commercials had to support that media. One of the naturals was cosmetic companies. They could really reach a woman where she lived (the pun intended) at home and in her heart of hearts.

The early and middle 1950s saw advertising extravaganzas in both TV and magazines and we became readily conditioned. Within no time we became accustomed to the two page advertising color spreads depicting the beautiful model and glamorous stars. We all wanted to look like them, and of course lipstick was always the biggest attraction, as well as the biggest seller. Their formulas were now steadily improving.

The turmoil of the 1960s with the unwanted Vietnam War,

with everyone feeling she could finally speak her mind, and conformity no longer the fashionable mode (as it was in the 1950s), makeup in general went every which way. Remember the pale lipsticks, the almost white and even white lipsticks we all wore? How unnatural and contrived we all looked!

The 1970s brought us individualism. We were appalled at our own government what with the Watergate affair, but cosmetics always being in step with the times saw that women wanted to do "their own thing" and Women's Lib was making its impact. We didn't have to emulate the stars anymore if we didn't want to, or be like anyone else—we could finally be ourselves. And so lipsticks became sheerer, more natural, regardless of their shade. Even dark lipsticks ranging all the way to brown were sheerer, and they appeared more natural and more sensuous.

Here we are looking toward the 1980s. Now most of the original cosmetic pioneers are gone and the companies have been taken over by huge pharmaceutical companies who perhaps run them with more integrity and less passion than before.

What's new about lipsticks? Well, there are always new colors— you can see that for yourself in the newspapers and magazines. But, to arrive at a really new look to make your lips more luscious and color more exciting, wear two lipsticks! Use any two lipsticks, regardless of their color, texture, or brand. They don't even have to be in the same shade range. Go ahead and experiment. Just for the fun of it, pick any two lipsticks on your dressing table with your eyes closed—you'll see, it works! (Except if you should happen to choose two really way-out, crazy shades.) This two shade technique is so simple it's almost silly and it is really the difference between just wearing lipstick and wearing LIPSTICK! You'll have women everywhere sauntering over to you to ask what shade of lipstick you're wearing (just as I do every day, no matter where I am).

Outline your lips with a lipbrush using the darker of the two shades and fill in the center with the lighter of the two shades. Then apply just a little clear lip gloss with the lipbrush to the center of the lips to blend it all together.

Now let me clarify one point. The darker outline should not be a hard grease line of color so that your lips are presenting two distinctly different shades. The outside edge of the outline should be clean and crisp but the inside should be unstructured as if you were applying one shade and hadn't finished filling in the center. Use the second lighter shade to fill in the center somewhat going over the first shade, but do not go near the outer edge. Now apply the lip gloss. The easiest way to do this so that the gloss will not make your lipstick bleed or feather is to pucker up as if you were going to blow a kiss and touch only the center of your lips with the gloss on your brush, smoothing it with the brush and keeping it well within the lipline.

Every woman will thus have her own exclusive shade of lipstick and you can't get more individual than that. Also, the depth of color this technique provides makes the color and texture look more interesting under any light! You can also get two extremely different effects. It depends on the order in which you apply them. By applying the lighter shade first to the center of your lips and *then* outlining with a lip brush using the darker shade, it will create a totally different effect than the one previously described. Both techniques work best if you lightly dust translucent face powder to your lips first and then apply the lipsticks.

These methods give your lips a special look that simply cannot be achieved with just one lipstick even if it were to contain striated colors, frost and gloss, all rolled into one. (That hasn't been done yet, but they're getting there.)

THE BETTER WAY TO BETTER LIPS

A lipbrush is a lipstick's best friend. If you have reached the age of 30 or over and have never used a lipbrush, I would like to convince you to try. Try this: Outline the upper lip from the center bow to right corner and then center to left corner, gently rounding the contour. Or, you may do it exactly in reverse, corners to center. On the lower lip draw a short straight line across the center at the lowest part of the lip, then gently curve the line to each corner. The brush offers accuracy, correcting the lipline more precisely, and easily shades one color into another. A sable brush with an even edge with the ferrule holding the bristles flat that is no longer than a quarter inch is the easiest and best. Make sure you always pick up enough color on the brush by brushing it back and forth against the lipstick. A brush may be cleaned merely by tissuing off the excess and if you wish, cleaning it every so often by dipping it into 70 percent alcohol and wiping dry.

Another useful cosmetic aid besides the lipbrush, which you might have even more confidence in using is a lip pencil. A creamy lip pencil (wood type) sharpened to a fine point, or one that has a sharp slant-edge (metal or plastic cylinder type) is very easy to use —even easier than applying lipstick directly from the tube. It offers the advantage of definite control to draw a more definitive line and the line will hold all day or all evening. This is especially helpful to women who complain about lipstick bleeding into vertical lines around the mouth. (In this case, be sure that the lip pencil is not too creamy and has a firm lead.) You can then fill in the rest of the lip area by applying color directly from the lipstick tube. Sound simple? It is! And, you'll love the results!

You may outline only your upper lip with either a lip pencil or lipbrush and color the lower lip using the age old method of smacking the lips together by rolling the upper lip over the lower.

Lipsticks not only color, but condition and protect the delicate tissue of the lips. Some formulations have built-in sunscreens for extra protection. A lip primer is a stick similar to a lipstick. It contains less wax and more emollients than the usual lipstick. It is used to further soften the lips and serve as a base for lipstick, making the lips shinier. But don't confuse this with lip gloss. They are two separate products, although a lip gloss may also be used as a base. (Some even have breath fresheners.)

Liquid lipsticks are not new—there are new revivals from time to time and they are on the market again. This time they are greatly improved so they may stay around for awhile. (They saw the height of their popularity starting right after World War II.) Heretofore, they were too drying to the lips and were unwieldy and messy to use. This is the main reason they fell into disfavor (besides, they leaked). Their current revival enjoys a creamier, shinier formula and a new convenience—they are packaged in leakproof automatic containers much like a roll-on mascara. They are especially convenient to use in a public place, particularly for adding gloss. (Other liquid lipsticks/glosses are packaged in roll-on applicators resembling a roll-on deodorant.) However, the main attraction as far as I am concerned is for the woman who is still an outline-holdout. She may very well like the automatic type with the sponge or felt-tip applicators or specially-contoured brush which provides an all-in-one convenience. It takes the place of lipstick, lipbrush or pencil, and gloss. In addition, it automatically dispenses a measured amount of the lip color. This control may be very helpful to those women who still refuse to use a lipbrush or pencil. In any case, for those who love to play with new gadgets (or who like nostalgia) liquid lipsticks are great fun.

Natural Lips for a Natural You

Always follow your natural lipline, even when making a corrected lip line. Every woman has natural curves to her mouth, so avoid pointed angular lines. However, the highest points of the bow should always be within the area that is defined and limited by the outer edges of the nostrils. When using a lipbrush, lip pencil, automatic lip color, or lipstick directly from the tube, maintain a closed, relaxed mouth. You may find you have better control if you rest your little finger on your chin with your elbow on the table or hold your wrist with your free hand. (See page 205.)

The Principle of Light and Dark Once More

Light colors enlarge the mouth; dark or tawny shades reduce.

CORRECTING A NOT-TOO-PERFECT MOUTH
TO REDUCE THE APPEARANCE OF A LARGE MOUTH

Stay within the lip line—cut the corners to a very narrow line of color. You may need a second application of your foundation before you powder, making sure each is dry. (The second coat may be blotted with tissue if time is of the essence.) Use subdued tones of darker lipstick shades and avoid bright, bright colors and light shades. Better yet, outline with dark shade and fill in with a tawny, lighter shade. Avoid frosted lipsticks and lip gloss.

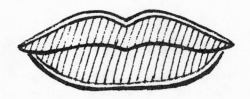

TO ENLARGE A TOO-SMALL MOUTH

Follow the natural lipline extending it about one-sixteenth of an inch (that's a hairline) over the lipline, or stay exactly on the lipline itself, rounding the curves to the corners. Balance the lips by extending slightly over the lower lip below the natural lipline. Use deeper shades for outlining and fill in with lighter, bright shades. Apply translucent lip gloss to both upper and lower lips.

TO PICK UP A DROOPY MOUTH

You will definitely need a lipbrush or lip pencil to lift outer corners of the upper lip. Draw an upward tilt, be it ever so slight, so no one suspects, but be sure the corners of the upper and lower lips meet exactly. Keep the fullness at the center of the lip.

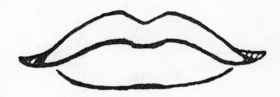

THIN LIPS

Outline with a darker shade of lipstick or lip pencil or even a soft light brown eyebrow pencil, ever so slightly over the bow of the upper lip and just slightly below the lower lip. Fill in with a lighter shade, making sure to fade the lighter color into the darker one. A bit of lip gloss on the center of both lips will make them look fuller.

THIN LOWER LIP

Extend the line of the lower lip ever so slightly over it. Fill in the lower lip with a lipstick that is several shades lighter than the upper lip but in the same shade family. This will equalize a thin lower lip with that of the upper.

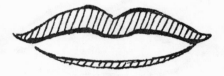

BRINGING A RECEDING LOWER LIP FORWARD

Use a darker shade on your upper lip and a lighter shade on the lower lip, but line the lower lip with the same darker shade very narrowly. Now, pucker up as if you were going to blow a kiss, and apply lip gloss to center of lower lip only.

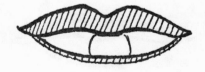

FULL LIPS

Outline the lips with a lighter shade, staying within the natural lipline. Fill in with darker shade. Pucker up as if you were about to blow a kiss and apply lip gloss, confiing it to a very small area in the center of the lips.

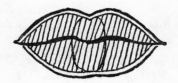

FULL LOWER LIP

Use lipbrush or lip pencil and stay within the lower lip line. Follow natural upper lip line. Apply gloss only to the upper center of lip.

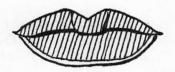

Artificial Light Drains Color, Daylight Accentuates Color

Decide what you are going to wear and let your garment be your inspiration in choosing your lipstick shade. It should be in harmony and flattering to both your coloring and your outflt, taking into consideration where you will be spending most of your time that day.

LIPSTICK SHADE GUIDE BASED ON
CLOTHING COLORS

Browns, beiges, yellows, greens — Lipstick should have an underlying gold tone

Blues and violets — Lipstick should have an underlying blue tone

Black or white — Choose lipsticks that are true, clear reds

Pinks, reds and oranges — Closely match or blend

LIPSTICK SHADE GUIDE BASED ON
YOUR EYE MAKEUP

No eye makeup — Use light pinks or corals or just lip gloss by itself

Minimum eye makeup — Use light pinks, corals, or soft reds

Daytime average eye makeup — Medium shades (lipgloss optional)

Daytime complete eye makeup — Any shade that has intenity of color, plus lip gloss

Nightime — More intense deeper shades ranging all the way to brown, plus lipgloss. Or use luminescent or frosted shades.

When it comes to lipstick shades, to be perfectly honest, all rules were made to be broken—if you know how! But everyone's teeth appear to be whiter by contrast with clear, true, medium reds. If your teeth have a yellow or orange cast, avoid orangey coral shades. If your teeth have a blue cast, avoid blue undertones, but if your teeth are grayish, a lipstick with a blue undertone will make them look whiter. Other than this, the world of lipstick shades is yours. But please remember one thing: Do not blot any lipstick until you are ready to eat or kiss.

Teeth

You could be the most beautiful woman, expertly made up, well groomed from head to toe, but if you smile and your teeth don't live up to the rest of you, the effect is ruined!

I have one admonition that should seem unnecessary to anyone over 30, much less to a teenager. Yet I find many women who should know better, using their front teeth to open bobby pins. Is this habit of opening bobby pins worth the risk of chipping a front tooth? Use the edge of the counter to open your bobby pins. The counter-edge saves your fingrnails too!

A professional cleaning at least twice a year is a must for the woman over 30, and should be more often for women who smoke. If there are more serious faults such as bad alignment, orthodontia is no longer the province of the teenager alone. Many of these faults can be corrected by wearing orthodontic appliances that are made of tooth-colored plastic rather than metal, and while they are not entirely unnoticeable, they are more aesthetically pleasing. Capping may be in order. Whatever the problem might be, see your dentist. It goes without saying that any missing teeth should be replaced with some type of bridge or denture as soon as possible, to prevent sagging facial muscles and to further prevent deep lines from forming around the mouth.

SOME OF US HAVE A DIFFERENT KIND OF PROBLEM

After we've brushed and flossed our teeth properly, after we've used our disclosing tablets and water pulsating devices such as a

233

WaterPik (even putting mouthwash right into its reservoir), after we've been checked out by our dentists twice a year and have been assured that our teeth are in good order, after they have been professionally cleaned with regularity, many of us have permanently stained teeth or inherently uneven colored teeth that no amount of toothpaste (or anything else) will make whiter and more even in color. Well, I have inside information that good news is coming. It shouldn't be too far in the future that our dentists will be able to cosmetically coat our teeth making them permanently whiter and more even in color. I know, many of us can hardly wait!*

---

* As we go to press, reports are coming in that there are quite a few dentists throughout the country who are now using this new technique with very successful results.

Last Words

YOUR ACCESSORIES

Even for daytime, don't forget your fragrance. This bit of mystifying allure makes all of us feel better. And whose spirits aren't lifted when some stranger (male or female) says, "Don't you smell delicious!"

While everyone is always inventing new places to wear fragrance, I still haven't found anything better than behind the ears, the hollow of the throat and the nape of the neck. True, there are other areas, but how can these traditional pulse points be omitted? Let me caution you not to wear fragrance when you know you are going to be out in the sun. Dabbing perfume behind your ears or on your neck before going into the sun can cause an irreversible condition of *retiform pigmentation* with some redness on the skin at the sides of the neck. It is almost impossible to treat, even by a dermatologist.

Today, more than ever, the ambience of fragrance is everywhere. We have all kinds of fragrances to choose from, for any time of day or any mood you happen to be in. Colognes are lovely for daywear and you can spray them into your hair for an even longer lasting effect. Toilet waters are somewhat heavier in strength than colognes and of course, perfumes are the maximum in strength.

France was the exclusive producer of fine, expensive perfumes for the last few centuries. (The art of perfumery has been around for some twenty-five thousand years; the word perfume comes from the Latin, meaning "through smoke.") It is only in very recent years that perfumes have been produced in America. Of course, we manufactured colognes and toilet water, but perfume is something new for us and now there are so many more to choose from. Use them for evenings—they're still not *that* inexpensive. Colognes and toilet waters of the same scent are a fraction of their cost that can (and should) be used lavishly as well as daily.

Also for daytime, don't forget your earrings. The gleam of silver or gold (real or otherwise) casts a very pretty glow on your face once you are made up. But remember, the glimmering type adds width to the face while a matte finish or dull surface will decrease width. Save the stones (real or otherwise) for evening.

MANNERS AND MAKEUP

A woman's concern with how she looks should be limited to the privacy of her own dressing room or the ladies room in a public place. There is almost nothing more distasteful to both men and women than observing a woman who makes a display of constantly checking or repairing her makeup in their presence. Then there is the type of woman who just can't pass by a mirror without casting anxious or admiring glances at herself (either she is completely unaware or thinks this fleeting behavior goes unnoticed). While it is actually deep insecurity, her conduct is interpreted as downright egotism which is anathema to most people. Such women are no longer beautiful no matter how beautifully they are made-up. "Set it and forget it" is a motto that reflects good breeding as well as good manners.

The reapplication of lipstick after one has eaten is the only acceptable cosmetic application in a public place. If there is need for anything more, a lady excuses herself to the ladies room and quickly takes care of her needs, making sure that the time spent there is unobtrusive to those waiting for her. I don't think any woman deliberately wants to be labeled egotistical or selfish.

A woman's appearance is a personal affair and should always be catered to in private. A truly beautiful woman is one who forgets herself and enjoys others so they can enjoy her.

HOW TO APPROACH A
COSMETIC COUNTER

To this day, I still employ a sort of little game I used to play when it was incumbent upon me to go into the stores to check if the beauty advisors or cosmeticians knew what they were talking about to their customers. Most of them did then and they do now.

I always played a little dumb, so I could successfully ask questions without arousing suspicion as to who I was or where I was from. I deliberately underplayed my own makeup or wore very little and appeared to be only slightly knowledgeable. I would ask questions designed to glean all types of information about an individual product, or a group of products. I found then, as I find today, that when you ask a question armed with a little knowledge —just quietly thrown into the conversation—if the lady behind the counter does not know or cannot answer your question, she will either go find out or will refer you to another salesperson who does.

You have the right to ask questions and receive satisfactory answers without feeling that anyone is going to browbeat you into buying more than you intended. If you know what you are after, you don't have to play dumb. It's your money and your face and it has been my intention to provide you with that needed knowledge. I once read words to this effect, "Americans always *think* they are right. The English *know* they are right." When you buy, *know* that you are purchasing the right product before you leave the cosmetic counter.

MAKEUP ACTION CAPSULES
(STEP-BY-STEP REVIEW)
DAYTIME COMPLETE MAKEUP

Cleanse. Wash eyes with eyewash. Use skin freshener (s) .

1. Moisturize face, throat, and neck. Apply eye gel (optional) .

2. Apply under eye concealer. Gently blend into lighter surrounding areas of your skin.

3. Apply your individual contouring (optional) with lighter shade concealer. (Note: if using highlighter or lighter shade of foundation, apply after your tinted foundation.)

4. Use dot or bottle method of applying your tinted foundation (see pages 160–161) . Use upward, outward strokes over entire face, throat, and neck, blending with your fingertips or dampened cosmetic sponge. Apply foundation so it is thin and evently distributed all over your face, but, very, very thinly on the eyelids. Blend right into your hairline, pay particular attention to nose crevices, laugh lines, around ear lobes, outward over jawline—go right over your lips. Continue under chin and down neck if you are not wearing a high neck garment. (If, on the basis of what you are wearing you want to omit neck area, do blend under chin.) Make sure there is no line of demarcation—fade edges to nothing.

5. Clean out corners of eyes and tips of nostrils with cotton swabs.

6. Apply blusher or rouge. Look into your mirror, smiling very broadly—make a really forced grin (it puffs out the cheeks) . Place a dot or two of color at the center of the most rounded flesh. Hold grin for a few seconds and start blending upward and outward almost to hairline, no higher than the top of the ear and no lower than the earlobe. Fade edges into hairline. Repeat on other cheek. Darkest portion of color should be at the center of your cheekbones or near the hairline, but subtly blended. Hollowing under the cheekbones is optional (see page 170) .

7. Apply any of the optional additional uses for blush or rouge (see pages 170–171) . Use sparingly and blend well.

8. Brush eyebrow hairs downward with your eyebrow brush. Use a sharp pointed pencil. (Note: if using eyebrow cake or powder, apply after face powder.) Start no further in than the inside corner of your eye. Curve the hairlike strokes to the peak and end no further than the outside corner of your eye, ending in a slightly upward tilt but always following your natural bone structure. Remove any excess or correct any mistakes with a cotton swab. Repeat on other eyebrow. (If needed, use folded paper method—see pages 105–106, page 175.) Now brush eyebrow hairs upward.

9. Allow foundation, rouge, and eyebrows to set for several minutes. Brush your hairline and arrange your hair. If more time is needed, put on your pantyhouse and bra, make the bed, return a phone call, etc. Just make sure your foundation is no longer tacky to the touch before proceeding.

10. Apply translucent face powder with clean powder puff or cotton using press and dust techniques (see page 182).

11. After selecting your eye shape (pages 186–199), gently apply eyeshadow of your choice in neutral colors. Allow eyeshadow to set for a moment and remove any excess with cotton swab.

12. Apply eyeliner of your choice starting at outside corner of eye and draw inward as close to the base of eyelashes as possible, refraining from going into the inside corner of the eye. Use blue-grey eyeliner to underline the eye starting at outside corner (if it applies to your eye shape). Repeat on other eye. If you use an eyelash curler, now is the time.

13. If you use supplemental eyelashes, apply them now (see pages 210–211 for technique). If not, apply mascara of your choice. Apply from roots to tips of lashes using two or three light applications, allowing each to dry before applying the next. If needed, separate the lashes with clean eyelash comb or point of a **Pick-A-Dent.**

14. Apply mascara to lower lashes (optional), first sweeping upward from underneath, then sideways, using the end or point of brush, then downward, separating and arranging.

15. Finish getting dressed.

16. Apply your lipstick, outlining with lipbrush or lip pencil according to your lip shape (see pages 228–231). For the two lipstick technique, see page 224. Apply lip gloss.

17. The final touch is optional—to set your makeup: Use cotton or a silk, natural or cosmetic sponge. Wring out in cool water and gently dab all over your face, throat, and neck. To further set eye makeup, use a cotton ball, moistened in cool water. Squeeze out almost dry and very lightly touch your eye makeup.

18. Use your favorite daytime fragrance and don't forget your earrings.

QUICK GETAWAY MAKEUP

*(Use Daytime Complete Makeup Action
Capsule for Techniques)*

Cleanse. Wash eyes with eyewash. Use skin freshener (s) .

1. Moisturize face, throat, and neck.
2. Apply loose tinted face powder or all-in-one tinted compact powder or matte finish foundation.
3. Apply powdered blusher.
4. Apply eyebrow pencil (if needed) .
5. Use eyelash curler (optional) .
6. If time permits, apply eye shadow and/or eyeliner.
7. Apply light coating of mascara.
8. Apply lipstick. If time permits, outline with lipbrush or lip pencil and apply lip gloss.

EVENING OR GALA COMPLETE MAKEUP

Use more vivid shades, including luminescents and frosteds. Your tinted foundation may be one or two shades warmer than your daytime foundation. For gala occasions, select your eye shadows to complement your gown (but not necessarily matching it) . Use supplemental eyelashes for more eye emphasis and glamour. When wearing low-cut dresses or gowns, blend foundation makeup down to your cleavage. And do cover over white strap marks on your back if wearing a backless gown.

1. Cleanse.
2. Wash eyes with eye wash.
3. Wipe face with skin fresheners.
4. Moisturize face, throat, and neck.
5. Apply wrinkle stick or eye gel (optional) .
6. Apply under eye concealer. Gently blend into lighter surrounding areas of your skin.
7. Apply your individual contouring with both lighter and darker shades. (See pages 144–150.)

8. Use dot or bottle method of applying your tinted foundation (see pages 160–161). Use upward, outward strokes over entire face, throat, and neck, blending with your fingertips or dampened cosmetic sponge. Apply foundation so it is thin and evenly distributed all over your face but, very, very thinly on the eyelids. Blend right into your hairline, pay particular attention to nose crevices, laugh lines, around ear lobes, outward over jawline—go right over your lips. Continue under chin and down neck. Make sure there is no line of demarcation—fade edges to nothing.

9. Clean out corners of eyes and tips of nostrils with cotton swabs.

10. Apply blusher or rouge. Look into your mirror, smiling very broadly—make a really forced grin to puff out the cheeks. Place a dot or two of color at the center of the most rounded flesh. Hold grin for a few seconds and start blending upward and outward almost to hairline, no higher than the top of the ear. Fade edges into hairline. Repeat on other cheek. Darkest portion of color should be at the center of your cheek bones, but subtly blended.

11. Hollow the cheekbones for a heightened dramatic effect. Suck in your cheeks and place a darker or brownish shade of blusher in the hollows, confining most of the color to that area. Use only the smallest dot of color and carefully blend one color into the other so there is no line of demarcation between the two shades of rouge. Blend the darker hollowing shade outward to the ear but not lower than the earlobe.

12. Apply any of the optional additional uses for blush or rouge (see pages 170–171). Use sparingly and blend well.

13. Brush eyebrow hairs downward with your eyebrow brush. Use a sharp pointed pencil. Use additional shades of gold or silver. (Note: if using eyebrow cake or powder, apply after face powder.) Start no further in than the inside corner of your eye, ending in a slightly upward tilt but, always following your natural bone structure. Remove any excess or correct any mistakes with cotton swab. Repeat on other eyebrow. (If needed, use folded paper method— see pages 105–106, page 175.) Now brush eyebrow hairs upward.

14. Allow foundation, rouge, and eyebrows to set for several minutes. Brush your hairline and arrange your hair. If more time is needed, put on your pantyhose and bra, return a phone call, etc. Just make sure your foundation is no longer tacky to the touch before proceeding.

15. Apply translucent face powder with clean powder puff or cotton using press and dust techniques (see page 182).

16. After selecting your eye shape (pages 186–199), gently apply eyeshadows in shades to complement your evening clothes. Allow eyeshadow to set for a moment and remove any excess with a cotton swab.

17. Apply eyeliner of your choice starting at outside corner of eye and draw inward as close to the base of lashes as possible, refraining from going to the inside corner of the eye. Use blue-grey eyeliner or a complementary shade for your evening clothes or gown to underline the eye starting at outside corner. If this technique does not apply to your eye shape, bring it in only ¼ inch from the outside corner of the eye. Repeat on other eye. If you use an eyelash curler, now is the time.

18. Apply supplemental eyelashes, using the technique on pages 210–211. Apply mascara to blend both the false lashes and your own together. For a gala occasion, tip the ends of lashes with gold or silver. Separate the lashes with the point of a **Pick-A-Dent.**

19. Apply mascara to lower lashes, first sweeping upward from underneath, then sideways, using the end or point of brush, then downward, separating and arranging.

20. Finish getting dressed.

21. Apply your lipstick, outlining with lipbrush or lip pencil according to your lip shape (see pages 228–231). For the two lipsticks technique, which is exceptionally great under night lights, see page 224 and use lip gloss.

22. The final touch is optional—to set your makeup. Use cotton or a silk, natural or cosmetic sponge. Wring out in cool water and gently dab all over your face, throat, and neck. To further set eye makeup, use a cotton ball, moistened in cool water. Squeeze out almost dry and very lightly touch your eye makeup.

23. Use your favorite perfume and wear your loveliest earrings, the more stones, the better. For your sake, I hope they are real!

Index

Accessories, 235–236

Acid mantle, 23–24, 59, 63

Acne, 28, 93–94, 121, 122, 166

Action capsule, 33, 238–243; for blackheads, whiteheads, and pimples, 99–101; daytime complete makeup, 238–240; evening (or gala) complete makeup, 240–243; eyebrow shaping, 109; meaning of, 8; for previously tweezed eyebrows, 104; quick getaway makeup, 240; three-minute nightly (step-by-step review), 84–85

Aging process: acceleration of, 29–30, 66; after 30 and being realistic, 1–6; attitude toward, 116–118, deceleration of, 64, 66–67; dry skin, 31, 67; heredity, 44, 118; oily skin, 38–39; sun, 28

Allergies, 123–126; hypo-allergenic cosmetics, 125–126; patch test for, 124–125

American Medical Association (AMA), 118–119, 205

American Society of Plastic and Reconstructive Surgeons, Inc., 117

Arden, Elizabeth, 222–223

Astringents: cleansing, 45, 60, 95–96; explanation of, 58–59; oily skin, 38, 40, 89; *See also* Skin fresheners

Bacteria, 126; hygiene, 51, 57, 102; in pores, 22, 92

Balance and harmony, 134–138; self-observation, 134–135; under eye concealers, 136–138; under makeup moisturizers, 135–136

Beauty salons, 150–151; special services, 108–109, 110, 112

Beauty tools, 19–20; brushes and sponges, 57

Birthmarks, 138

Black women, 38, 39, 119; profiles, 39–41; special notes, 41–42

Blackhead extractor, 95; sterilizing, 96–97

Blackheads, 24, 33, 91–92; action capsule, 99–100; dealing with, 94–96; extracting, 97–98

Blood vessels: cold and hot water, 54–55, 88; eyes, 57; skin structure, 15, 22, 88

Blusher or rouge, 168–173; common mistakes, 169; other uses for, 170–171; purpose of, 169; shade guide, 172; types of, 172–173

Bone structure, individual contouring for: cheeks, 170; eyebrows, 174; eyes, 200–201; face shapes, 150–157; noses, 139–147

Bronzers, 29

Brown liver spots, 119–120, 137–138

Capillaries, 119–120; broken, 120; how to conceal, 137, 166; shock or trauma, 88

Chemical face peels, 121

Chins: chin straps, 115; double chin, 149; and foundation, 159–162; and

243

powder, 178; protruding, 148; short, 143; receding, 142; undue strain, 29

Cigarette smoking, 26

Cleansing, 43–70; action capsule, 84; discipline, 69–70; of eye makeup, 215; eyes, 57–58; moisture and moisturizers, 45, 50–52, 61–65; precleansing, 44; with rinsable cleansers, 49; with skin fresheners, 58–60; skin type and, 40–42; soap and water, 47–56; stroking motions, 45–46; supplementing your skin program, 85–90; tissuing-off, 46–47

Cleansing cream or lotion, 44–45; moisturizing ingredients of, 45–46; nighttime, 65–69

Collagen and elastic fibers, 28, 29–30, 114

Colognes, 235

Complexion brushes, 51

Concealers, cover-ups and highlighters (under eyes), 136–138

Contact lenses, 216–217

Contouring, 138–150; daytime, 138–143; nighttime, 144–150; principle of, 138

Cosmetic counter, how to approach, 237

Cosmetic language, 8–9

Cosmetic surgery, 116–119

Cryosurgery, 120–121

Cysts, 93

Daily cleansing procedures and products to use, 71–83

Daytime contouring, 138–143; broad or flat nose, 140; deep smile lines from nose to mouth, 141; frown lines between eyebrows, 141; heavy jawline, 142; long nose with center bump, 139; long nose with high bridge, 140; long or pointed nose, 139; receding chin, 142; short chin, 143; short flat nose, 140; vertical lines from mouth to nose, 143; wide nostrils, 141; See also Nighttime contouring

Dead skin cells, 85–86; definition of, 7; epidermis, 7, 63, 66; exfoliation of,

86; renewing cycle, 23; shedding, 51

Dentists, 233–234

Depilatories, 110–111; 112, 122

Depilatron, 112–113

Dermabrasion, 121

Dermatologists, 9; and acne, 93–94, 121; and allergies, 123–124; and moles, 120; and warts, 120; when to consult with, 28–29, 37–38, 42, 48, 50, 93, 98, 110, 123, 167

Dermis, see Epidermis and dermis

Directory of Medical Specialists, 118

Dressing table, 16; beauty tools for, 19–20

Dry skin, 36; cleansing, 41; See also Ultra-dry and Very dry skin

Electrolysis, 112–113

Emollients: in eye and neck creams, 67; ingredients in cleansing cream or lotion, 44; in lipsticks, 227; in moisturizers, 62, 63; in night creams and lotions, 65–66

Environment: and blackheads, 91, 94; and heredity and life-style, 44; and moisturizing protection, 62–64; and sleep, 66; and soap and water, 47

Epidermis and dermis, 21–22, 28

Evening and gala makeup, 241

Exfoliation, 42, 120; products to use, 86

Eye creams, gels and wrinkle sticks, 67, 136

Eye drops, 57–58

Eye makeup, 184–199; to appear almond shaped, 187; beauty rule for, 186; bringing out deep-set eyes, 188; bringing out shallow eyes, 189; bringing wide-set eyes in closer, 190; to contour flat lids for rounder look, 198; contouring slanted eyes, 195; diminishing prominent lids, 194; disguising heavy folds over outer half of upper lids, 196; disguising older eyes, 197; disguising overhanging upper lids, 196; to dramatize light-colored eyes needing more depth, 191; elongating horizon-

INDEX

tally narrow eyes, 193; elongating round eyes, 192; to enhance "large" wide-set eyes (and bring them closer together), 190–191; to lighten dark eyelids and correct corner shadows, 199; and lipstick shade guide, 232; to make eyelids more prominent, 198; minimizing protruding round eyes, 192; to open squinty eyes or narrow eyes, 193; picking up droopy, sleepy-looking eyes, 195; playing up small eyes, 188; reducing bulges below the brows, 197; reducing puffiness, 199; shaping well-proportioned large eyes, 194; under eye concealers, 136–138; widening close-set eyes, 189

Eyebrow shaping, 105–107; action capsule, 109; the arch, 106–107

Eyebrows, 173–177; coloring, 108–109; and electrolysis, 108; penciling, 174–176; powdered makeup, 176–177; shade guide (pencil or powder), 177; tweezing, 101–104

Eyeglasses, 215–220; face shape and, 217–219; sunglass frames (color guide), 219–220

Eyelash curlers, 206–207

Eyelashes: care of, 207–208; powdering, 180–181; supplemental, 209–214

Eyelid surgery (blepharoplasty), 117–119

Eyelid tissue, cleansing, 215

Eyelids, powdering, 180–181

Eyeliners and eyelining, 203–204; brush care, 206; and false eyelashes, 205–206; and mascara, 208; removers, 206; shades for, 204; types of, 206; underlining, 205

Eyes: blinking, 202; care of lashes, 207; extra dry spots, 67, 167, 168; squinting, 26, 219; washing, 57

Eyeshadow, 200–202; shading and blending color lesson, 201–202; types of, 200–201

Eyewash, 57

Face lift (rhytidectomy), 29, 117; temporary, 116

Face shapes and hairstyles, 150–157; diamond shaped, 155; heart-shaped, 154; long, oblong or inverted triangle, 156; round, 152; square, 153; triangular, 157

Facial exercise and massage, 29, 113–114, 117

Facial flaws, 119–121; major, 119–120; minor, 120–121

Facial hair, 109–113

Facial saunas, 42, 88–89

False eyelashes, 209–214; caring for, 213; eyeliner and, 205–206; individual, 214; removing, 212; technique for, 210–211; that really look false, 213–214; types of, 212

Fibrin foam technique, 122–123

Food and Drug Administration (FDA), 108, 122, 131

Foundation (base), putting different type products together with, 133–135; See also Tinted foundation

Fragrances, 235–236

Freckles, 121, 167

Frownies, 115; See also Glabella

Glabella, 115

Glands: adrenal, 111; eccrine, 23–24, 63; pituatary, 111

Hair follicles, 111; and electrolysis, 112; and eyelashes, 207; pores, 23, 91; sebaceous glands, 23–24; tweezing, 101, 104

Hair removal, 109–113

Hairstyles and face shapes, 150–157

Health, 13–14

Heredity, 44, 118, 120

Hirsutism, 112

Homemade cosmetics, 126

Keloids, 42, 119–120

Keratin, 23

Labeling, cosmetics, 124–125; astringents, 38; rinsable cleansers, 49;

soaps, 47; sunscreens, 27
Lighting, 17; day and night lights, 130,
   150, 158; and foundation, 158–159,
   162–163; and lipstick, 225, 231; and
   powder, 178; and wrinkles, 65, 89
Lip pencil, 226–227
Lipbrush, 225–226
Lipgloss, 224; at bedtime, 69; and lipstick, 133, 224, 227, 232
Lipstick, 221–232; balance considerations, 225; bringing a receding lower
   lip forward, 230; to enlarge a too
   small mouth, 229; for full lips, 231;
   for full lower lip, 231; historical
   background of, 221–224; liquid or
   cream, 227; naturalness, 227–228; to
   pick up a droopy mouth, 229; principle of light and dark, 228; to reduce appearance of a large mouth,
   228; shade guide based on clothing
   colors, 231; shade guide based on
   eye makeup, 232; for thin lips, 230;
   for thin lower lip, 230; two-shade
   technique, 224–225

Magnifying mirrors, 16–18
Makeup, 129–243; accessories, 235–
   236; action capsules (step-by-step
   review), 238–243; after cosmetic
   surgery, 119; awareness and morale,
   130; balance and harmony, 134–138;
   bedtime, 69; blusher or rouge, 168–
   173; complete re-do (in the evening), 130–131; contouring, 138–150;
   eye, 184–199; eyebrows, 173–177; and
   eyeglasses, 215–220; eyeliner and
   eyelashes, 203–214; eyeshadow, 200–
   202; face shape and hairstyles, 150–
   157; foundation (putting different
   products together), 133–135; good
   balance in, 15–16; know-how, 14–15;
   lipstick, 221–232; list of essentials,
   19–20; and manners, 236; manufacturers, 131–132; and pores, 15, 62,
   63; powder, 178–183; as protection,
   26, 30; time in making up, 215;
   tinted foundation and how to buy,
   158–168

Manners and makeup, 236
Manufacturers, 131–132; commercial
   vs. homemade, 126; industry image
   and quality control, 3; products, 71
Mascara: applying, 208; and false eyelashes, 213; shade guide, 209; types
   of, 208–209
Masks, 38, 42; products to use, 87–88
Mature woman, products for, 89–90
Melanin/melanocytes, 25, 120; black
   women, 39
Menopause and post-menopause, 111,
   113
Menstrual period, 94
Moisture and moisturizers, 61–65, 129;
   brands to use by skin type, 71–83;
   and moisturizing, 61–62; oily skin,
   38; primary purpose of, 62–65;
   tinted, 135–136; under makeup,
   135–136
Moles, 119–120
Mustache, 110, 113, 138

Neck: and blusher and rouge, 171; and
   cosmetic surgery, 113, 118; creams,
   67; exercise, 114; and foundation,
   159–164, 167; and fragrance, 235;
   and moisturizing, 61; and powder,
   167, 182; and sebaceous glands, 39,
   62
Night creams and lotions, 65–69; extra
   dry areas, 67; man in bed and, 68–69
Nighttime makeup, 130–131, 158; action capsule, 241–243; broad or flat
   nose, 146; contouring, 144–150;
   double chin, 149; heavy jawline, 148;
   hump nose, 145; long nose with high
   bridge, 145; long or pointed nose,
   144; long, pointed nose with center
   bump, 144; one side fuller than the
   other, 145; prominent temples with
   high forehead, 150; protruding chin,
   148; protruding upper lip, 149;
   sharp upturned nose or bulbous tip
   between nostrils, 147; short, flat
   nose, 146; wide bridge, 147; wide
   nostrils, 146; See also Daytime contouring; Eye makeup; Gala

Normal combination skin, daily cleansing procedures, 73–82; products to use, 73–76; profiles, 31–36

Noses, 135, 137; and blush, 168, 171; contouring, 139–141, 144–147; and powder, 179

Oil (sebum), 23–24, 31, 38, 62

Oily skin, 33; cleansing, 40; facial saunas, 89; and foundation, 158, 166; products to use, 72–73; special note on, 38–39; throat and neck, 62

Opticians/opthalmologists/optometrists, 214

Oriental women, 119

PABA (ingredient), 27

Perfume, 235–236

Photosensitivity, 29, 235

Pill, the, 28–29

Pillows, 66–67

Pimples, 92–93; action capsule, 100–101; alternative method for dealing with, 98–99; dealing with, 94–96; extracting, 97–98

Powder and powdering, 178–183; dust method, 182; eyebrow, 176–177; eyelids and eyelashes, 180–181; press method, 182; special notes on, 167–168; tinted, 180, 182; translucent or transparent, 182–183; virtues of, 180–181

Precleansers, 44

Product lists, 72–83

Puffiness, 67, 137

Resorcinol, 38

Revson, Charles, 223

Rouge, see Blusher or rouge

Royal College of Physicians and Surgeons of Canada, 119

Rubefacients, 59

Rubinstein, Helena, 223

Scars: acne, 121, 122; keloid, 42, 119; and makeup, 138; moles and warts,

120; plastic surgery, 119; skin tags, 121

Sebaceous (oil) glands, 23–24, 31; blackheads and whiteheads, 94; and neck, 62, 67; and pimples, 93

Shade guides: blush/rouge, 172; eye makeup for individual shapes, 187–199; eyebrows, 177; eyeliners, 204; foundation, 165; lipstick, 231–232; mascara, 209; sunglass frames, 219–220; tinted moisturizers, 135–136

Silicone, 122

Skin fresheners, 58–60; brands to use by skin type, 78–86; ingredients, 59; use of, 58–59; water and, 59–60

Skin structure, 21–30; effects of sun on, 25–29; epidermis and dermis, 21–22, 28; oil glands, 23–24; preventive care, 29–30

Skin types, 31–41; black women, 38, 39–42; dry, 36; normal combinations, 33–35; oily, 33; oily sensitive, 38; selecting products for, 71–90; ultradry, 37–38; use of soap and water, 47–49; very dry, delicate, 37; very dry, delicate with oily patches, 37

Soap and water, 47–56; brands to use by skin type, 72–83; debate over, 52–56; interviews with women, 49–50; skin types and, 47–49; virtues of, 47

Sun, effects of (on skin structure), 25–29, 39; sunscreens/sunblocks, 27; sunscreens/sunblocks in foundations, 165

Sunglasses, color guides for frames of, 219–220

Sweat pores, 23–24

Tap water, 59–60

Teeth care, 233–234

Tinted foundation (base), 158–168; applying, 159; blending, 159–160; buying, 162–164; liquid or cream foundation (base), 133; reason for wearing, 158; shade guide, 165; special notes on, 167–168; tech-

niques of, 160–162; texture, 158–159; types of, 166–167
Tissuing-off, 46–47
Translucent powder and liquid or cream foundation, 180
Tweezing eyebrows, 101–104; action capsule, 104; additional notes on, 103–104

Ultra-dry (dehydrated) skin, 37–38; cleansing, 41; products to use, 82–84
Ultraviolet rays, 25–29
Under eye concealers, 136–138; liquid or cream foundation (base), 133
Under makeup moisturizers, 135–136

Vasoconstrictor eye drops, 57

Very dry (sensitive, or delicate) skin, 37; cleansing, 41; products to use, 80–82

Warts, 119–120
Whiteheads, 92; action capsule, 100; dealing with, 94–96; extracting 97–98
Witch hazel, 40
Wrinkles: chin straps and frownies, 115; cosmetic surgery, 116–119; dermabrasion and chemical face peels, 121; eye area, 67; increasing and creating, 26–28, 66, 114; preventing, 26–28, 66–67, 87, 219

X-ray therapy, 119